JOSEPH COVINO JR

STAY FIT (AND HOT) FOR LIFE:

A WORKOUT PRIMER

EPIC PRESS

DEDICATION

For the misled Youth, guided gullibly like so many innocent lambs to their ritual slaughter, so severely and so tragically astray

ACKNOWLEDGMENT

This is creatively and interpretively an original work of nonfiction based partly but not entirely upon the bodybuilding, fitness and health principles of Steve Reeves as put forth in his definitive work, Building The Classic Physique—The Natural Way. All direct quotes directly attributed to Steve Reeves are hereby referenced from Steve's book unless otherwise annotated, partly or fully quoted, or paraphrased from other alternate sources as cited from the printed mass media. All material originating from Steve Reeves is rightly attributed to him. All other material originates from the writer of this book and is directly attributable to myself.

CONTENTS

PREFACE:

TRAIN—DON'T TALK—FOR RESULTS

"He(Steve Reeves)was the most beautiful human to ever walk the sand of Muscle Beach."— Harold Zinkin, the first Mr. California

Ever since running track during my senior year in high school I've kept up to the present day a fairly regular and rigorous physical regimen consisting mostly in the past of calisthenics, running, stretching and swimming. Roughly a decade after graduating, though, a tribute–paying retrospective on Steve Reeves appearing in the May 1983 issue of *Muscle & Fitness* magazine motivated me to take up weight training in a most enthusiastic but uninstructed way, making extremely limited use of a generous neighbor's very basic barbell set. Inspired by Steve's powerfully informative interview and profile—in which he voiced and revealed at least small but significant facets of his vast store of bodybuilding knowledge(like recommended reps, sets and speeds of specific exercises)—I made the most of the least learning. Insight gleaned exclusively from an incomplete magazine interview—as educational and enlightening as it proved to be—was naturally sketchy at best. My resultant weight training workouts then were respectable enough but in the end quite mediocre in both quality and substance—to say nothing of notably deficient in producing any noticeable muscular growth. Later on my neighbor with the weights moved away(as well I did myself)and for years afterwards, discouraged partly by my failure to make much conspicuous progress in my muscular development, I regrettably lost both my energy and enthusiasm for bodybuilding.

With publication of Steve's complete and comprehensive bodybuilding book—***Building the Classic Physique: The Natural Way(1995)***—my resolve to devote myself seriously(and strenuously)to mastering the art and science of real bodybuilding with real passion and zeal was renewed anew! So thanks to Steve

Reeves there I vigorously strove in my early 40s, throwing myself once more with might and main(not to mention sweat and strain)into mightily intensive weight training—with, I must modestly boast, swift and astonishing results! And I didn't even get my hands on Steve's book until roughly January 1997 after reading Steve's interview with George Helmer in a 1996 issue of *Cult Movies* magazine. Now I only regret Steve didn't publish it decades earlier so that my younger muscles could've reaped its incredible benefits—though muscles of any age can incredibly benefit!

Once I did get hold of Steve's book I decided to practice his *"Championship Workout"* as correctly and precisely as I possibly could, following exactly his suggested workout schedule and paying close attention to such details and particulars as breathing, grip placement, method of movement, positioning of the body and limbs, rest periods, training order—everything. Next I wrote down on separate blank index cards(which went along with me on every trip to the gym)every single exercise scheduled in the workout—each in their proper order—including descriptions of their correct form and style. As a helpful and reassuring reminder I put down on yet a separate index card Steve's basic bodybuilding principles of *"Maximum Muscular Development."* Then I set about taking great pains to perform them—painstakingly!

Few though those basic principles may be: when followed to the letter as I've followed them they really do work—quickly and with astounding effect! Remarkably revealing was Steve's slowed–down, deliberately resistant rep speed—especially on the lowering or negative parts of exercise movements—and experiencing that wonderful *"momentary muscular failure."*

Finally I felt I had found real and natural body-building! Nobody(and I mean nobody!)at the gym where I worked out trained Steve's way—the right way! And in a very humbled way—since his work-out schedule forced me to train using lighter weights with deep concentration in perfect form and strict style—I felt truly sorry for so many others training so outwardly hard while making so little and limited bodybuilding headway, typically because they cheated themselves out of their own growth and development by bouncing, jerking, swinging and otherwise cheating on their exercises. So if you think there's no such thing as a *"right"* way of doing things there's usually a better way—and Steve's way is *BEST!*

Ever since I was a youngster going with wide-eyed wonder to Saturday movie matinees I had most certainly always aspired to look something like my childhood hero and motion picture film idol, Hercules, though I hardly ever dreamed it could actually be at least somewhat possible. After all, what kid who ever saw Steve's magnificent, perfectly proportioned and symmetrical image up there on that spectacular silver screen—whose *"athletic fantasies,"* as the magazine profile put it, were *"fueled"* by his cinematic mythical portrayals—didn't aspire to look like him? But it is actually possible! And after putting Steve's truly effective bodybuilding principles into actual practice for a relatively short time I am actually beginning to look something like Steve—or, rather, roughly how he used to look at age *17!!!*

Never could I be more pleased and grateful to Steve and his incomparable book for the great bodybuilding ground I've gained in so short a time. To this day the natural classic physique I've been blessed to build for myself owing solely to the knowledge acquired from Steve's phenomenal book still leaves me spellbound— and ever anxious and eager to get to my next work- out—often being barely able to wait out my rest days off from training due to the amazingly rapid and vis- ible strides I make during each and every workout.

"It is my contention," Steve heartened us, "that every man, regardless of his size, can so develop his body as to rate the envy of the folks too lazy, or per- haps not sufficiently interested—to do something about it. I say that we cannot help the way we are born—but we certainly can help what we do with the body we are born with."(*Dynamic Muscle Building*, Page 50).

This modest fitness book is my devoted tribute to Steve Reeves and what he has done for me and what he can do for you and so many countless others should they resolve simply to embrace and benefit by Steve's timeless knowledge and wisdom. Resolve to thorough- ly study and learn from Steve's marvelous book and I guarantee that you too can build and develop your own truly classic physique—the natural way!

FOREWORD:

WHY RELY ON REEVES FOR VERVE

"I've been told that 'there's going to be some backlash from the bodybuilding community as a result of your strong words, Steve.' My response to this charge is: 'Who cares?'"—Steve Reeves

STAY FIT FOR LIFE is the personalized dedication the late, great bodybuilding legend, *STEVE REEVES*, wrote on the title page of the complimentary copy of a hardback edition of his book for which I had done some equally complimentary proofreading: *Building The Classic Physique—The Natural Way*. Admittedly I inserted the parenthetical(*AND HOT*)phrase to somewhat sensationalize the title of my own Reeves–inspired fitness book even if the subject–matter contained herein is anything but sensational. In fact the matter in hand couldn't be more serious and compelling: at a time of life when many men my age(50–plus)are dreading their supposed declining years or advanced age this modest and unassuming bodybuilding book written by Steve Reeves quite literally transformed not only my physical body but my entire outlook on life by infusing me with new life and exuberance, thoroughly rejuvenating and reinvigorating me with youthful vim, vigor and vitality—correctly, safely, effectively, naturally—and without harmful resort to dangerous drugs, chemicals or other unnatural so–called health supplements.

My own fitness book, on the other hand, describes in detail how I've adapted and applied the health and fitness principles of Steve Reeves to my own life and physical exercise regimen—and explains why you should perhaps adapt and apply them to your own as well for your own best benefit. It aspires by interpretation only to supplement—not supplant—Steve's masterly bodybuilding book in its hopefully original perspective and presentation. Also, it imparts my own personal prescription and tricks of the trade, so to speak, for staying fitter, healthier, stronger, more energetic, vital and alive than ever. No one can predict with absolute certainty how long much less how fit or healthy they'll live, but with informed, intelligent and knowledgeable training you can most definitely energize, invigorate and vitalize your life by strengthening the quality of your health and fitness regimen. If knowledge is power, as they say, then my book can empower you just as Steve's book empowered me to not only defy age and physical decline but also to defeat them for the longest possible period. "You can't outrun the Grim Reaper!" a friend of negatively gloating *San Francisco Chronicle*(8 June 2003) staffer, Kim Severson, would yell at joggers from cars. Perhaps. But you can most assuredly **RETARD** the Grim Reaper!

"A person simply cannot live fully if he is not healthy," Steve astutely observed. "He can have money, fame, friends and influence, but still he will only be partially alive if his health is under par...None of us know what the future holds in store; fortunes can be lost, friends can move away and be seen no more, power can vanish, but good health if properly cared for is a substantial thing, a platform upon which a tower can be built; a tower which can be fortified as a protection against any unexpected emergency."(*Dynamic Muscle Building*, Pages 161–162).

Quality—not quantity—is what Steve's superlative method of bodybuilding, health and physical fitness training is all about. That translates quite simply into setting balanced goals which marry(not divorce)bodybuilding and fitness, which in turn when met produce real and observable results(both felt and seen)in terms of both enduring muscle and muscular endurance—whether aerobic or anaerobic. In a nutshell that means attaining the best and most results in the least time.

STAY FIT(AND HOT)FOR LIFE

"Doing something beats doing nothing" is a typical but stupid sentiment captioning an equally stupid "fitting in fitness" article written by staffer Susan Fornoff for the *San Francisco Chronicle*(19 January 2003). But if your training is detrimental, ineffective by way of real results or even harmful—if, in short, it lacks quality—then you're not only wasting both your time and effort but risking serious or permanent bodily injury as well. In that event you'd be better off doing nothing indeed!

Lately not one but two matron writers for the same paper hit their readership with a double–whammy–of–a–promotion—both(8 June 2003)a full–fledged "health–and–fitness" article and book review—promoting, so to speak, yet another self–styled fitness "expert" and "science" writer for the *New York Times*, Gina Kolata, who's on a cross–country jaunt promoting in turn her recently published "layman's"–science book about "exercise and conditioning." Kolata, wrote *San Francisco Chronicle* staffer, Carolyne Zinko, doesn't "want to appear to be some sort of exercise guru in gym togs on the jacket of her fifth book." Well, not to worry—there's quite honestly no threat of that. At 5–foot–3 and 115–pounds she's sickly and drastically underweight for any sized bone structure. And at just 55–years-old her baggy eyes, lined face and saggy neck together conspicuously display all the tell–tale signs of premature aging. None of these factual and forthright(if unflattering)observations are meant to be maliciously critical but such a person whose exercise regimen obviously doesn't work for them simply shouldn't be play–pretending in public to be some fitness "expert"—no matter how many molecular biology or mathematics degrees she has nor how many stationary "spinning" bikes she pedals! Even if she pedals at 13 miles–per–hour, which I seriously doubt, cycling is an inferior aerobic activity in terms of calorie–burning potential compared to swimming, running or even Steve's own power–walking.

"She(Kolata)writes that muscles use fat and carbohydrates as energy sources," Zinko reports. If so, then the puffed–up and over–praised "Pulitzer Prize finalist" has evidently failed to do her proverbial homework if she overlooks that other crucial energy source: *glycogen*(like fat a *stored* form of energy).

Kolata challenges the "maximum heart rate" for monitoring exercise intensity(speed or exercise workload), according to Zinko. If so, then she's got her terminology wrong for a start—it's *"maximal"* heart rate, which contrary to what Kolata insinuates isn't some arbitrarily set percentage at all but rather an ample range of 60 percent to 90 percent accounting for relative light, moderate and strong exercise intensities. And the 220–minus–age formula(for computing "target or training heart rate")Kolata disputes has an admitted "variability of plus or minus 10 to 12 beats per minute(*Durstine&Pate*, 1993)"—not the 30 beats that Kolata exaggerates.

Kolata questions the so–called "fat–burning zone," according to *San Francisco Chronicle* staffer, Kim Severson, "that mythical notion that exercising slowly burns more fat than working out more vigorously. Pure garbage, she says." Not entirely. Kolata's just drastically behind the times! Nowadays the "fat–burning" benefits of different types of exercise(aerobics in particular)is most often discussed in terms of caloric cost, which pertains to energy expenditure. And yes, the caloric or energy output cost of walking is comparatively less than that of jogging or running owing to slower speeds(intensities), though the caloric cost of Steve's power–walking(at intensity speeds of five miles per hour or faster)can indeed approximate that of jogging or running. Granted, caloric or energy cost increases proportionately with increased intensities or speeds. But the caloric or energy cost per mile is roughly the same for different people running and jogging the same mile at relatively faster and slower speeds. You needn't be "blinded by science" to appreciate that simply targeting your distance is just as critical as targeting your intensity(speed)and time. So briskly–paced walking at greater distances over longer periods of time can be as equally beneficial health–wise and weight–wise as jogging and running less distances at faster speeds. Not to stray too far from the true point in dispute: carefully and cautiously consider the source once confronted with any self–styled fitness "expert!"

In this fitness book I've concisely distilled Steve's most critical concepts and precepts for you to incorporate and profit by in your own personal exercise regimen. Strictly observe Steve's style of training and, I guarantee you, you'll never, ever waste even a millisecond of your time or effort working out at the gym or anyplace else! No training style is set in stone, carping critics and detractors might spout. Well, the Steve Reeves natural classic physique and how he built it *is!* Like Steve I tell it to you straight! Sometimes I resort to strong language to put across my points and get through to the reader but never get put off by that. Bear with me and bear in mind that my sole purpose in writing this book is to encourage you to avail yourself to the fullest of Steve's supremely sage knowledge and wisdom. Again I guarantee you that should you take full advantage of Steve's acutely astute fitness, health and training advice you'll never, ever regret it!

And if by chance you don't like my book then don't ask me to alter it to suit your style or taste—like Steve then my "response" will only be: write your own bloody book!

ONE:

PHYSIQUE CRITIQUE

"If you have fully developed shoulders, a tight midsection that displays abs, and have good calves, I guarantee you are going to have a physique that will turn heads!"—Steve Reeves

STAY FIT(AND HOT)FOR LIFE

In the familiar television infomercial for the supposed "best home gym" called "Bowflex" self–styled "Trainer to the Trainers"(I don't know who else but himself conferred on himself that title), Tom Purvis, quite pompously introduces the company's Vice President of Marketing, Randy Potter—stripped down(body–sprayed)to his red gym shorts—to demonstrate the machine like this: "This is what every guy wants to look like! Right? Guys! You wanna look like Randy? Well, listen up!" Preposterously implying that Randy's physique is "proof" of the contraption's supposed effectiveness.

Well, Tom, listen up: **WRONG!** Randy's nothing like I'd want to look—ever! Nor are you, for that matter! First off, Randy suffers from a bodily disorder afflicting many men who train with weights but still have disproportionate physiques: comparatively underdeveloped lats(back)and legs.

Likewise, in the infomercial for the Weider "Crossbow" machine host, Chris Leary, introduces another self–styled "fitness expert," David Sinclair, this way: "I may be stating the obvious here but it looks as though you know a little about fitness. Am I right there?"—alluding presumably to Sinclair's moderately muscular biceps(arms)—to which Sinclair retorts with a smirk: "A little bit. Yeah."

A teeny–weeny little bit, judging by Sinclair's hump-shouldered rhomboids(upper back muscles)and stick–thin legs, which even his knee–length short pants cannot conceal!

Before jumping then so rashly to so silly to say nothing of so insulting a conclusion, Tom, carefully check this out:

In the opening title sequences of the French–Italian major motion picture film, *Giant of Marathon(1959)*,

23

Steve Reeves as the Greek Olympiad champion, Phillipides, strikes impressive and imposing poses in various positions of active athletic prowess—javelin–throwing, swimming, shot putting, wrestling, striding, riding upon the shoulders of his compatriots and receiving his laurel wreath of victory—all displaying his picture–perfect physique.

Listen up, Tom, and mark me well: that's what I want to look like—or even something like that or anything even remotely comparable to that. Even a distant approximation of that would surpass looking like Randy by interstellar light years! Getting to look like that won't ever be attained by using a "Bowflex," so sell it to the gullible! Get my drift, Tom?

§

STEVE REEVES as a world–class bodybuilder quite unequivocally pioneered and perfected the greatest, most magnificent and matchless *NATURAL CLASSIC PHYSIQUE* of all time—the like of which the world had never before seen nor will ever see again. He ardently believed in the absolute beauty and value of a fully–developed physique that's balanced, proportioned and symmetrical. "I would recommend that a person have a symmetrical, classical type physique," Steve told George Helmer in an interview for *Cult Movies* magazine. "It's more desirable to the general public, although a few fans like that extreme bulked up steroid type physique. I'm glad more people are getting into the sport."(Number 18, 1996, Page 43). He won every single major bodybuilding title of his day, including Mr. America(1947), Mr. World(1948)and Mr. Universe(1950). Even though he gained great fame and fortune portraying mythical heroes like Hercules in some 14 Italian sword–and–sandal films throughout the 1950s and 1960s his first love and truest passion always remained bodybuilding and training to build his natural classic physique. "At times," David Gentle wrote of Steve for *Natural-Strength.com*, "Reeves gained or lost muscle tissue almost at will, yet always retaining a harmonious and balanced physique. Never did one feature lag behind or outshine another."(30 June 2000). Ron Avidan wrote for the *Almanac of Men's Bodybuilding*: "With his perfect physique and flawless symmetry, Steve Reeves made the phrase 'V Taper' a popular phrase in bodybuilding." Jan and Terry Todd wrote for the *Gale Encyclopedia of Popular Culture*: "Few historians would argue with the premise that no bodybuilder before or since Steve Reeves has ever had such a truly classic physique."

Just what exactly is a natural classic physique? It's a physique that's as fully developed, perfectly balanced, proportionate and symmetrical as possible. By proportionate Steve meant that the neck, biceps(arms)and calves of the legs should measure exactly the same in size. So the natural classic physique bodybuilder strives to build and develop broad, squared shoulders with wide, V–shaped lats(back), slender hips and waist with everything else in perfect proportion. Our primary purpose for going to the gym to train and work out should necessarily be to build and develop fully a physique which is as pleasingly balanced, proportionate and symmetrical as humanly possible. Balanced proportion and symmetry then should be the overriding driving forces motivating all our bodybuilding training. "When one comes into a gym to build a classic physique," Steve wrote for *All Natural Muscular Development* magazine, "they should not be concerned with simply adding size for the sake of adding size or in lifting heavy weights simply for the sake of lifting heavy weights. You must have a purpose or a reason for your training and that reason should be tempered with only one word—*PROPORTION*. There must be training logic applied to your endeavors."(February 1998, Volume 35, Number 2, Page 128).

§

Now that we've established what our first and foremost training objective should be let's consider briefly why striving for balanced proportion and symmetry is superior to trying so vainly to build and develop sheer size(bulk or mass)and/or strength for their own sake alone.

Obviously, we're all born with different genetic potential and no two human bodies are exactly alike physically. So the all–important question yet to be posed is: how do we set a balanced standard for muscular mass that will be equitable to everyone and still be proportionate and symmetrical?

Really the answer's quite simple: since we all have a bone structure that's mostly proportionate to our height, for each person we should base our utmost potential proportions and symmetry upon our individual height and bone structure(size). If our body size and weight excessively surpass our God–given height and bone structure then our body functions less effectively and less efficiently. So once we surpass that weight which is most ideally compatible with our height and bone structure our body not only becomes disproportionate and unsymmetrical but functions less optimally as well.

That's why most if not all contemporary physique

bulk–builders, as I term them, simply cannot run, jump and play along with classic physique bodybuilders. "Or," Steve wrote for *All Natural Muscular Development* magazine, "they'll fall victim to training their strongest or best body–part to bizarre and downright freakish dimensions—but at the expense of what they should be concentrating on with their training—symmetry and proportion."(February 1998, Volume 35, Number 2, Page 178). Because they've divorced real bodybuilding from true fitness to such an extreme degree, their disproportionate and unsymmetrical body size and excessive weight make optimal functioning with what I call their cockeyed Popeye physiques physically impossible. From a strictly health and fitness standpoint, that's a profoundly undesirable state of being.

"I think the ideal weight would be based upon height," Steve elaborated, generally defining the bodybuilder's ideal height/weight ratio for *Flex* magazine. "Let's say a person is six feet tall, then he should weigh about 200 pounds. As you progress each inch over six feet, you should add 15 pounds. If you're 6'1", then you should weigh 215 pounds; if you're 6'2, you should weigh 230 pounds, and so on. If you're under six feet, you should drop 10 pounds(from the base of 200)for every inch of height you are under six feet. If a person is 5'11", then a good muscular weight for them would be 190 pounds. I was 6'1" and weighed 215 pounds, and it seemed ideal for me."(Page 113).

Refer in Steve's bodybuilding book to his Classic Physique Height/Weight Proportion Chart to precisely calculate your own individual ideal classic physique height and weight.

§

Body–Building V. Bulk–Building
(Good Quality Muscle V. Poor Quality Muscle)

So you think you want to train to become some bloated, out of shape, poorly conditioned, short–winded titan? In a few words: a round–shouldered, hump–backed, turtle–necked, alligator–abed bulk–builder. In a word: *BIG!* If so, I earnestly urge you to seriously reconsider for the sole sake of your own health, fitness and best benefit.

To begin with we can distinguish between real bodybuilders on the one hand and bulk–builder pretenders on the other:

Most bulk–builders might command sufficient anaerobic energy to perform certain feats of strength at high intensities for brief periods of time. On the superficial face of it they may look fit, healthy, muscular and strong yet they're sorely lacking in one crucial thing—the aerobic capacity to cycle, run, stretch and swim for prolonged periods of time. In reality, then, these big, over–bloated bulk–builders lack inner endurance and—much like premature ejaculators—fizzle out real fast. At the opposite end of the fitness spectrum are highly conditioned, in super–shape long–distance and marathon runners who command abundant aerobic capacity but who lack that muscular, strongly–built look. In reality, most world–class marathoners look gaunt, gangly and emaciated.

Natural classic physique bodybuilding, quite contrary to contemporary bulk–building, combines and strikes a healthy balance between these two extreme tendencies to build and develop both enduring muscle and muscular endurance. So you can forget right off that unmentionable profiteering jester out of New York who body–types everybody as a cone, hourglass, ruler or spoon! Notice he doesn't strip off his shirt during his infomercials to show how his fitness system works—or doesn't work—for him. Attaining true health and fitness then demands: muscular strength, muscular endurance and aerobic capacity.

Finally, we can distinguish between training to build good quality muscle and bulking up with poor quality muscle to achieve sheer size alone simply to look *"big."* Always opt to build up with good quality muscle over bulking up with poor quality muscle. Good quality muscle is built, developed and gained solely by means of correct training in conjunction with all–natural nutrition and supplementation. Poor quality muscle is added by gaining weight and fattening up your muscle tissue through the inferior medium of ingesting artificial and unnatural growth–inducing substances like anabolic steroids—without which those so–called "muscles" quickly shrink like rapidly deflating tires. As he proudly told *Smithsonian* magazine, Steve "never used any of these chemicals, like steroids, that weight–lifters use today. It's too bad how they bloat themselves up. When your arms begin to look bigger than your head, something is wrong."(November 1998, Volume 29, Number 8, Page 136).

All things considered, pursuing our ideal image of a fully developed physique comes down in the end to coming to a correct conclusion about whether bodybuilding is superior to bulk–building—or whether building balanced, quality proportion and symmetry is superior to bulking up for bloated, mis–proportioned mass—in terms of true health and fitness, and committing ourselves to a correct course of action for achieving precisely what we conceive.

Maybe you misguidedly think that by getting *"big"*

and amassing mis–proportioned mass that you're going to attract attention to yourself, overawe people and command or inspire respect when in reality most objective onlookers will likely gawk at you like you're some kind of freak of nature—with revulsion—rather than marvel at you with admiration.

What makes contemporary bulk–built physiques inferior to classic body–built physiques is precisely their conspicuous lack of balanced proportion and symmetry: necks, arms and calves which are mismatched in size together with overgrown trapezius muscles which afflict contemporary bulk–builders with their round–shouldered, turtle–necked deformity. Worse still, they lack any distinctive individuality. Since they mostly train the same, do the same routines and ingest the same synthetic supplements it's really no surprise that they mostly look the same—like clones cast from the very same bulk–builder mold! "How can you express your own unique, individual potential?" Steve questioned for *All Natural Muscular Development* magazine(July 1997, Volume 34, Number 7, Page 104).

The bottom line is: mis–proportioned, misshapen mass does *NOT* a balanced, proportioned and symmetrical physique make!

"Once a person exceeds his ideal weight for his height," Steve wrote for *All Natural Muscular Development* magazine, "he becomes out of proportion and not only no longer possesses a 'classic' physique, but doesn't function optimally either."(February 1998, Volume 35, Number 2, Page 178).

TWO:

SENSIBLE WEIGHT TRAINING

"I feel that the often used saying, 'No pain, no gain' is a negative slogan and should be replaced by a more positive approach of 'No brain, no gain.' Be a thinking bodybuilder."—Steve Reeves

Iput it more bluntly than ever polite Steve: train smart(with brain), not stupid(with pain)! If doing strength resistance training with weights ever inflicts pain upon you or any part of your body then you're doing something radically wrong and should immediately stop doing it—no matter if even the current "Mr. Olympia" himself is trying to impose it upon you! So don't ever be what I call a dumbbell–**DOPE** by letting some bulk–builder force you to feel a "burn" in your muscles while performing any strenuous exercise. If you do feel that intense burning sensation("burn")in your muscles while working out then take heed and *STOP*—it means extreme fatigue due to overexertion and a tip–off from your nervous system, cautioning you against increased risk of injury to your muscles or connective tissue(tendons in particular). Stay smart then and lessen the intensity level of whatever movement is inflicting pain—or "burn"—on your muscles!

When working out, Steve Reeves believed in following a certain sensible training **LOGIC**.

"I figured out a better way to train," Steve told *Flex* magazine, "more scientifically. I'm a logical man, and my method, which I learned...was to work one muscle group until it was depleted and then move on to the next. That's when I made big progress." Against all logic, reason, rational thought and good sense, however, you'll still see people in gyms beating their brains out—not to mention the rest of their body parts—clinging stubbornly to harebrained, haphazard training routines just to create the self–deluding illusion of working out. "You have to be a thinking bodybuilder," Steve stressed. "You can't just go by somebody else's routines—there has to be a method, a logic to your training."(*Dynamic Muscle Building*,

Page 39). Just going through the motions of working out is a royal waste of your time and effort and amounts to what I term: ineffectual movement without substantial result.

§

Two MAJOR Training Traps(And Their Proponents)To Avoid Like The Plague

·Aping Like A Mindless Monkey A Bulk–Builder At Your Gym. Parroting at your gym some bulk–builder(who's perhaps won some trophies at amateur competitions perpetuating standards as mis–proportioned as the physiques on parade)may pander to his ego—at your own expense—but will do next to nothing to help you build and develop your own classic physique. Bear in mind what David Gentle wrote for *NaturalStrength.com*, "Physiques are as ever influenced greatly by judging requirements and of course, beauty is in the eye of the beholder."(30 June 2000). Unless of course your perceptions are completely warped like those of Randy Shandis, the "Filthy Critic," who reviewed Gladiator the movie for *BigEmpire.com*, spouting that actor "Russell Crowe is a hell of a lot better looking than Steve Reeves." He ought to christen himself as the *IDIOTIC* critic instead! Thinking then that your gym's resident bulk–builder must know what he's doing or talking about simply because he happens to be "big" is equally misguided and will get you next to nowhere so far as building and developing your own classic physique is concerned. Why? What works for a bulk–builder will not necessarily—and most likely never will—work for you! In all likelihood, it will in reality prove to be quite harmful to you by virtue of detrimental movements and piss–poor training habits if anything. Blindly emulating the dictums and licking the feet of a bulk–builder like a lapdog is a surefire formula for real bodybuilding failure! Ineffectual movement without substantial result! "It seems to me that too many people just follow somebody else's dictates blindly," Steve wrote for *All Natural Muscular Development* magazine. "They'll see somebody with big arms and they'll do the routine that this individual utilizes—not that his program will necessarily work for them."(February 1998, Volume 35, Number 2, Page 178). Cable television's ESPN channel exercise program, *Body–Shaping*, features **Rick Valente**— the only currently prominent bulk–builder I've seen teaching correct, slow–and–smooth weight–training techniques. If you give credence solely to bulk–builder instruction, then by all means check Rick out!

•**Cheating Yourself By Cheating On Your Exercises**. Cheating usually assumes the form of bending, bouncing, jerking, rocking, swinging, tilting and twisting either the body or the weight to lift excessively heavy weight which you're incapable of lifting in perfect form or strict style—instead of truly isolating the body part or muscle group meant to be worked. If such cheating were at all advisable then the activity could be called weight–bouncing or weight–swinging rather than weight–*LIFTING*. When you flout perfect form or strict style just to handle heavier weight you cheat only yourself since you deprive your muscles of stimulation they need to grow bigger and stronger. All you ever maintain or retain by cheating is what I term a static—or unchanging—physique. Doubling or even tripling poor quality training still produces only abysmal results. *HOW* you exercise, train and work out is eminently more important to building and developing a truly dynamic or spectacular physique than what exercise you do or what weight you lift. Cheating is just another type of ineffectual movement without substantial result! "Their training sessions were marked by a new level of discipline," official biographer, Chris LeClaire, wrote of Steve's early workouts at Ed Yarick's Physical Culture Studio in Oakland, CA in 1946. "While lifting, they tolerated no bouncing of the weights, no cheating of any kind and held their Golden Rule: 'If you cheat, you cheat yourself!'"(Page 56).

§

Smart Dos and Stupid Don'ts of Weight Training

The Golden Rule: To build maximum muscular development lift the maximum weight you are able and ready to lift in perfect form or strict style—meaning performing your repetitions *SLOWLY AND SMOOTHLY*—without bouncing or swinging the weight to create centrifugal force or momentum.

Smart Dos of Weight Training

•**Check Your Ego At the Gym Door**. Training by Steve's techniques takes abundant patience, persistence and perseverance.

•Set specific goals to match correct training techniques: build mainly strength by doing five to six sets of near–maximum lifts for two to three repetitions, resting up to five minutes between sets. Build a combination of strength and muscular growth by doing five to six sets of near–maximum lifts for five to six repetitions, resting for two to three minutes between sets. Build maximum muscular development and growth by lifting the maximum weight you can handle with perfect form or strict style—doing three sets of eight to twelve repetitions, resting only 45 seconds to one minute between sets or the time it takes only one workout partner to perform one set.

•Warm up thoroughly with five minutes of aerobic exercise and some stretching before each and every workout, or at least until you break a sweat.

•Train your body by body part or muscle group in this exact order: deltoids(shoulders), pectorals(chest), lats(middle and upper back), biceps(front arms), triceps(back arms), quadriceps(front thighs), hamstrings(backs of legs), calves, lower back, abdominals(midsection), neck. In other words, work the smaller muscles of your upper body first and work down last to the largest and strongest muscles of your lower body—your legs. Train the muscles where the blood logically flows—downward and backward with(not against)gravity—since you logically pump blood(carrying oxygen and nutrients)to those muscles being worked! When you work against gravity you needlessly stress your system. "Some people," Steve affirmed, "believe that building the body is an art, others that it is a sport, and others think it's a science. My own opinion is that it is more of a science, and that's why the body must be trained in a specific sequence in order to obtain optimum results." Steve recalled for *Iron Game History* the methodical and systematic training style he practiced during his youthful "Muscle Beach" days: "I had a certain routine I did and I'd use a pulley for this, I'd use a bar for that, a dumbbell for this and a barbell for that. I liked order and I liked to have everything the way I wanted it, so I could follow the sequence I wanted."(December 2000, Volume 6, Number 4, Page 5).

•Number the repetitions you perform by your

muscle fiber type. If you have fast–twitch muscle fibers then perform five to seven repetitions for each
set. If you have slow–twitch muscle fibers then perform 12 to 15 repetitions since you can maintain your
level of exertion for longer periods of time without tiring due to your greater endurance capacity. Dispar-
ity in muscle fiber types is simply another significant
reason why bulk–builder techniques likely won't work
for you.

•Adjust your weight poundage by your height and
bone structure and what your muscles can handle
with utmost efficiency. Start your set with your top
weight. Retain the same weight or lower it slightly
with each set. "What I do is this," Steve advised. "I
use a weight that I can use for eight repetitions. When
I reach 12 I add five pounds and start again at eight,
and work up to 12. After repeating this for a month or
two, you will be surprised to see how much you have
increased the weight used on the exercise."(**Dynamic
Muscle Building**, Page 81).

•Train your muscles with deep concentration
through their fullest possible range of motion which
your articulations or joints(not someone else's joints)
will permit—meaning complete contraction and complete extension in perfect form or strict style—to get
every last rep from every last set performed. Carefully avoid doing incomplete or what I term halfway,
half–baked, half–arse movements! "When I worked
out," Steve recounted, "I'd concentrate exclusively on
the muscle being worked. I'd concentrate on the movements, doing them nice and slow so that I could feel
the movement all the way up and all the way down.
I used a full range of motion and it really worked out
well for me...I have always approved of working the
muscles completely, through their entire range of ex-

tension and contraction. I feel that this gives the physique long lines of flowing muscles. Short movements tend to bunch up the muscle masses. Some bodybuilders may like a 'knotty' type of development. I prefer the more classical, flowing lines."(***Dynamic Muscle Building***, Pages 13, 154).

•Be broad by training wide with wide–grip exercises: wide–grip behind–the–neck presses for the shoulders, wide–grip bench presses for the chest, wide–grip behind–the–neck chins for the back.

•Breathe throughout your repetitions: Inhale(take in and hold your breath)at the point of greatest effort or exertion. Hold in your breath until you pass through the halfway or midway point of the movement. Exhale(let out your breath)at the completion point of the movement. In other words: Breathe in just before the positive part of the movement, hold your breath halfway through the positive part of the movement, breathe out through the negative part of the movement. Bench press example: breathe in deeply as you lower the bar to your chest before you press it up. Hold in your breath through the halfway or midway point of the positive(hardest)part of the bench press. Breathe out at the topmost point or negative part of the bench press. "Remember," *Muscle&Fitness* magazine(30 June 2004)quoted Steve as suggesting, "to be most effective and to aid in the development of the thorax, the breathing should be full and deep throughout the exercise."

•Perform the positive(concentric)part of the movement in two seconds. Perform the negative(eccentric) part of the movement in three seconds. Concentrate deeply as much on the negative as on the positive part of the movement. "Now you can eliminate it(momentum with free weights)by going slow, but who

does that?" spouts self–styled "Trainer to the Train-
ers," Tom Purvis, during the "Bowflex" infomercial.
Who does that? Who does slow negative repetitions?
Steve Reeves did. I do. You should too.

•Perform eight to 12 repetitions lifting the most
weight you can do in perfect form or strict style. Perform five to seven repetitions lifting heavier weight.
Perform 12 to 15 repetitions lifting lighter weight.
Lighten your weight if eight repetitions are too difficult. Raise your weight if 12 repetitions are too easy.
Perform 20 to 25 repetitions for calves and abdominals.

•Pause a beat between repetitions at the top of the
positive(concentric)movement before performing the
negative(eccentric)movement.

•Perform three sets of three exercises for each
muscle group. Diversify your training by doing three
sets of two different exercises for each muscle group
or two sets of three different exercises for each muscle
group. If your time is extremely limited circuit train
by doing only one set of one exercise from top to toe
for each body part or muscle group without any rest
between sets. "I have found three sets of each exercise
suits me best," Steve recounted. "Less does not pump
up the muscles enough, while more tends to make
the muscles stale and they cease to grow."(*Dynamic
Muscle Building*, Page 155).

•Rest two minutes between sets. Rest three to
five minutes between training different body parts or
muscle groups.

•Intensify your training by shortening your rest
time between sets and muscle groups.

•Stay standing and keep your body in motion between sets by pacing or shifting your weight from foot
to foot. I often do calf–raises in place by raising up on

my toes.

•Perform all movements with perfect form or strict style, deeply concentrating on isolating the specific muscle fibers being worked. Cheat only on your last repetition once your muscles experience momentary muscular failure(fatigue)and cannot do another strict repetition. "I maintain a strict exercise form always," Steve stressed, "using as heavy a weight as I possibly can. This style suits me best, for I like to feel and fight the weight at all times."(**Dynamic Muscle Building**, Page 154).

•Perform each and every set all—out or until your muscles experience momentary muscular failure(fatigue).

•Train no more than 2–1/2 hours during any single training session or workout. "If you train long, chances are you're going to have to keep something in your energy gas tank and not give it all you've got each set, just so you can make it through that long workout," Steve wrote for *All Natural Muscular Development* magazine. "That's spreading your effort of intensity over a long period of time. Not the most intense way to train. Try decreasing the amount of time in the gym and increasing the amount of effort you put into each rep, set and exercise. When it comes to high intensity training, longer isn't necessarily better."(December 1997, Volume 34, Number 12, Page 128). "What you need to have in order to build muscle is a well balance of intensity and duration," Steve elaborated. "If the intensity of your training is too high, you can't workout long enough to build maximum muscle size; but if the intensity of your training is too low, you can go for long duration but you're not getting any benefits because it goes on and on and on—you're wasting your time. It's a waste of time unless you have the right balance of intensity and duration and a good rest period for recuperation."(**Dynamic Muscle Building**, Page 16).

•Train no more than three days per week on alternating days(Monday, Wednesday, Friday or Tuesday, Thursday, Saturday). "Listen to your body," Steve wrote for *All Natural Muscular Development* magazine, "and only train it when it is completely recovered from your last workout and all the soreness is gone."(March 1998, Volume 35, Number 3, Page 196). "When you're working your various muscle groups," Steve elaborated, "you're also working your nervous system because you're concentrating hard, you're under the stress of trying to get that last rep in and, of course, the stress of the actual workout. If you do this every day or more than three times per week, neither your muscles nor your nervous system has time to recuperate. However, if you train(as I advise)only three times per week, you don't have to worry about your nervous system being drained as your whole body is given sufficient time to recuperate—and even gets stronger, allowing you to come to your next workout loaded with energy and enthusiasm."(**Dynamic Muscle Building**, Pages 16-17). "The reason I don't believe in working out every day is that, even if your muscles aren't taxed by such training, your nervous system is—especially if you're training as hard as you should; i.e., with full concentration and giving that last rep your absolute maximum effort. Obviously, you can't give it that 100 percent effort every day, as your nervous system has to have sufficient time to relax, calm down and regenerate, just as your muscles do. You must bear in mind that when you work out, it's not just your muscles that you're training; you're also training your mental attitude and your nervous system."(*Dynamic Muscle Building*, Page 116).

•Drink plenty of water with electrolytes(chloride, potassium, sodium)throughout your workout.

•Learn to effectively ignore the ignorant in gyms by turning a deaf ear to and tuning out the limitless stuff and nonsense about training which you'll commonly hear or overhear in gyms—because you'll get an earful enough of it and then some to spare! With just 45 seconds to rest in–between your sets you've got scant time for socializing anyway. "And I didn't want to be bugged when I was working out," Steve harked back to his youthful "Muscle Beach" days for *Iron Game History*. "I wanted to do my routine in a certain period of time. I'd be happy to talk to somebody before my workout or after my workout if they wanted to know something—my ideas about bodybuilding, what they should do or whatever. I'd be happy before or after. But during, that was a no–no."(December 2000, Volume 6, Number 4, Pages 5-6).

Stupid Don'ts of Weight Training

•Don't over–train by training more than three days per week. You stimulate but tear down muscle tissue when you train. You rebuild and develop muscle tissue when you rest. Muscle tissue recovers, recuperates and grows when you rest. You lose muscle tissue when you over-train. You cannot put out your utmost effort with over–training. "The people who have to worry about over–training are the ones that will spend one–to–two hours a day, six to seven days a week, engaged in what they mistakenly think is bodybuilding training," Steve wrote for *All Natural Muscular Development* magazine. "While such training may stimulate their muscles, they do not allow sufficient recovery time to elapse in order for the growth that they've stimulated to take place."(August

1997, Volume 34, Number 8, Page 104). "And make no mistake," Steve elaborated, "rest is just as important as working out. A lot of bodybuilders don't have much—if any—recuperation periods factored into their weekly workout schedule, with the result that they don't grow much muscle. They work out, and work out, and work out, and work out again; with each workout draining their muscles—with no time for recuperation and growth. These bodybuilders are actually tearing down more muscle than they are building!...A lot of modern bodybuilders exercise twice a day, six days a week. With such a program, when do you have time to recuperate? The answer is that you don't have it! And, if you're going to do that, you can't be giving your all(two workouts a day, six days a week)to your bodybuilding workouts, because it wouldn't be possible. You just couldn't...The same thing applies for those guys who train twice a day, six days a week. They can't be giving their 'all' because it's impossible to give your 'all' that many times per day, that many days a week without holding something back. Eventually their training becomes stale and they start to hate their workouts instead of enjoying them."(*Dynamic Muscle Building*, Pages 16-17).

    •Don't demonstrate that you're an amateur by posing and flexing your "pumped up" muscles in front of the mirror during your workout when in reality you're breaking down—not building up—muscle tissue.

    •Don't obsess over how "big" you're looking—or not looking. Proper proportion in your physique will naturally make you look "big" no matter what your stature. In short, don't let yourself get afflicted with the disorder called muscle dysmorphia or reverse anorexia now more commonly known as: ***BIGORE-***

XIA—typically manifested by constantly checking yourself in mirrors and constantly comparing your physique with other physiques to measure up to them! I've watched you do both so you know you're guilty!

•Don't obsess over how much weight you're lifting. Your purpose for going to the gym is to build and develop—not demonstrate or display—muscle size and strength. Aspire to improve rather than impress. While you're attempting to impress someone else is improving! If you're awestruck at some bulk–builder at your gym bench–pressing upwards of 300 pounds, or more, don't get overexcited; and let me assure you that no world record in power–lifting is in danger of being broken there since world–class power–lifters bench–press double that poundage and more! "A muscle works harder when it's made to work in a strict range of angle and motion," Steve wrote for *All Natural Muscular Development* magazine. "Sloppy form and heavy weights don't do much except impress your friends and get you injured. Think not about the amount of weight used, but rather, how you can make the muscle work harder."(December 1997, Volume 34, Number 12, Page 128). So keep complete control of your own weights. Don't let the weights—just inanimate objects, after all—control you! For that matter, don't let anybody else—especially some amateur bulk–builder—try to control you, either, by browbeating or bullying you to lift weights you're not yet conceivably capable of lifting!

•Don't over–develop the trapezius muscle at the base of your neck unless you want to be afflicted with the bulk–builder's round–shouldered, turtle–necked bodily deformity. "In building the classic physique," Steve wrote for *All Natural Muscular Development* magazine, "it is important that the trainee shy away from exercises that stress muscles such as the trapezius muscle at the base of the skull, because the bigger the traps are, the narrower your shoulders will appear. Instead of a square–shouldered look, a person with overdeveloped traps looks round–shouldered."(February 1998, Volume 35, Number 2, Page 128).

•Don't over–develop your midsection's oblique muscles unless you want your waist to look wider and so detract from your broad–shouldered classic physique look. "Another thing to avoid is training the oblique muscles of the midsection," Steve wrote for *All Natural Muscular Development* magazine. "If you build these muscles up too much, they will also detract from your broad–shouldered appearance and make your waist wider."(February 1998, Volume 35, Number 2, Page 128).

•Don't train with more than one workout partner. A perfect rest period is the 45 seconds to one minute it takes your workout partner to perform one set. Training with more than one workout partner is both inefficient and ineffective since your muscles cool down too much while you're waiting your turn to do your set. "We all know the effects of what happens when you rest too long between sets; the muscle loses its pump and many times, the level of intensity can't be recaptured again until the next workout," Steve wrote for *All Natural Muscular Development* magazine. "The key is to rest just long enough to catch your breath and keep the muscle pumping, while the blood is still concentrated in the muscle you are working. Don't let the muscle fully recover until you are out of the gym!"(December 1997, Volume 34, Number 12, Page 128). "Of the nine total sets that I did per body-part," Steve elaborated, "each of those sets were performed 'all–out' and with just enough time in between each set for my workout partner to grab the apparatus, or the weight, and hit it. In other words, I trained with very high–intensity; with very little rest in between sets—just enough rest to do the exercise properly and to let the other person do his afterwards. I found that having one workout partner was ideal—but if you have more than one person, you ended up resting too long and your muscles would cool down too much in between sets. If you don't have a workout partner or prefer training alone, you should rest just long enough in between sets as it would take if somebody else was going through a set of the same exercise. In other words, figure out how long it takes you to do your set, say, 45–seconds, and then rest about the same length of time."(Dynamic Muscle Building, Page 43).

•Don't train with weight too heavy for you to handle. When you lift overly heavy weights your connective tissue(tendons)—not your muscle—tends to take over the work, grow and get strong instead of your muscle. "I know a lot of guys over the age of 50," Steve cautioned, "who are walking around with bad knees, bad hips and bad backs because they tried to use too much weight too soon when they were working out—or they didn't take the time to warm up correctly—or both."

•Don't plop yourself down onto a bench while waiting for a workout partner to do their set. Learn and perform stretches specific to the muscle groups you're working in–between your sets. Steve stretched his lats following his one–arm rows, for instance. "I'd go over to the squat rack," he wrote, "grab the horizontal support bar, pull back and down to stretch my lats— it always felt great after a hard lat workout to stretch them out immediately afterwards."

•Don't drop the weight during the negative (eccentric) part of the repetition. *Resist* the weight instead.

•Don't stupidly "blow the weight away from you." Inhaled oxygen is needed to energize the muscles being worked. Exhaled oxygen only mis–serves to deprive those muscles of both oxygen and the energy essential to work. "And oxygen," Steve observed, "as we all have been taught in early grammar school days, is absorbed by the blood stream, thus producing energy. Naturally, the greater absorption of oxygen, the greater the benefits to the entire blood stream, and the greater potential energy in the body."(**Dynamic Muscle Building**, Page 61).

•Don't use a perilous—and unproductive—thumbless grip while doing your bench presses. Should your bar roll out of your grip during your bench press you could break your sternum bone.

•Don't settle into a workout "routine" where you're simply repeating the same monotonous movements over and over, time and time again. "For instance," Steve explained, "I don't believe in keeping the same routine all of the time. In fact, I don't even like to call a workout a 'routine,' I prefer to call it a *schedule*.' A 'routine' means doing the same thing over and over and over again. What I like to do is change my *schedules*."

•Don't "spot" your workout partner by assisting with the lift of the weight, which doesn't permit your partner to experience momentary muscular failure(fatigue)on their last repetition. Assisted repetitions may be a cute kind of male bonding but they mis–serve only to hurt rather than help your partner's progress. A helpful "spotter" simply counts your repetitions and lifts the weight once you experience momentary muscular failure(fatigue)so you can focus and concentrate on completing your last repetitions.

•Don't blurt out silly and senseless sayings like *"C'MON! It's all you!"* which mis–serve only to break your workout partner's focus and concentration while spotting since they should pretty much already know full well they're the only person lying supine upon the bench beneath the weight.

•Don't ridiculously demand of your training partner downright impossible feats of strength or added repetitions after a max–out set. As Steve asserted, "A training partner should be able to know when to encourage you and when to shut up."

§

Weight training and working out are **NOT** about the painful, pressure–filled and unproductive **DRUDGERY** of irrationally fast, frenetic movements or stressful strain and tension. They're meant to energize and empower—not debilitate, demoralize or unnerve—you. Quite the contrary, they're supposed to stimulate, invigorate, refresh and even **RELAX** you. Fatigue and tire you, **YES**. Hurt and pain you, **NO, NO, NO, NO!!!!** Training should be something **PLEASANT** which you look forward to and **EN-JOY!**—not dread!

"Always remember," Steve emphasized, "that exercising should tire the body but should be relaxing—refreshing to the mind and nervous system. And that to get the most benefit out of an exercise it is important that you do it correctly." **REAL** bodybuilding, he affirmed, "properly performed—is not about stress and negativity but positive, good old–fashioned hard work."

"I would like to impress upon you," Steve reiterated, "that all these exercises...for the development of the body, are merely the means to an end; the end itself can be reached only by hard work—by the diligent application of the means used to achieve the desired results. Wishful thinking won't do it. Complete knowledge of the proper exercises won't do it. But actually doing those exercises regularly WILL give you the body development you want...Keep in mind that it takes work—and a lot of it! And, equally as important, it takes patience and determination...I would like to remind you...that only by patience, and diligent devotion to the actual work involved, can ANY real development be achieved."(**Dynamic Muscle Building**, Pages 54, 64).

Work is a four letter word but it's hardly a dirty word. Training that produces real results is neither more nor less than simply **WORK**—but never, ever pain!

Painful Postscript

In his article for the *San Francisco Chronicle*(4 May 2003)titled, "Going Navy," staffer Christopher Heredia recounted a perfect instance of ineffectual pain–inflicting movement without result with his pain-filled report about a supposed "Navy SEAL boot camp class" at Crunch Gym in San Francisco painfully conducted by "instructors," so–called, Sev Kristofich and Derek Nicholas.

Even before any "exercise" commenced, Kristofich reportedly "chided" his class for not "stretching while he was explaining some of the routines." For that matter, any instructor worth his SEAL salt would've dutifully and responsibly instructed his students in correct stretching techniques in advance.

"We're going to work off each other's energy,"

Kristofich reportedly lectured. "The result is you're going to do more than you've previously done or ever thought you could do." All anybody's likely to do in this instance is "work off" the hot air spouted by an overblown blowhard who thrives on hearing himself talk(and yell).

"We're here to get a lot of results because I'm gonna whoop your ass," Kristofich reportedly blustered. "People shouldn't take this class unless you want to get worked. Giving up or sticking to where you are with your workouts is why you look the way you do."

Getting real results from getting worked is one thing. Getting your butt "whoop"–ed by some loudmouth is why looking the way you do likely won't transform much less improve.

"It has to do with your percentage of body weight and the number of reps," Kristofich reportedly preached. "As we go on, the reps get heavier. This will get you cut."

Your body weight might feel "heavier" as your reps get harder but doing frenetically fast reps with half–baked movements and sloppy form won't ever "get you cut"—doing as many slow and smooth reps as you can in perfect form and strict style will!

"You think you can't change, you can't do anything. Well, you're stuck in a negative impact zone," Kristofich reportedly negatively proselytized.

Yeah, well, if you throw good money after bad(and worse)following fitness shysters you'll just get stuck fast in a negative and static no–development zone physique–wise.

"At the point of fatigue," Kristofich reportedly sermonized further, "where you think you can't do one more rep, is that crucial moment where you're on the cusp of getting results...That's why when people get tired in the class I try to get 'em pissed off, so they can work off their anger."

You're "on the cusp" of getting yourself hurt and injured, quite the contrary, once you let some shyster force you to worthlessly perform movements beyond fatigue without rest—during which real "results" occur. Intensify your training instead by simply shortening your rest periods between bouts of correctly executed movements.

Heredia's pandering piece features a photograph of "instructor," Derek Nicholas(replete with ear piercing and tattoos), applying "pressure" from above to some unsuspecting "student" dupe performing push-ups stressfully positioned with his upper back bowed over and his lower back lopsidedly dipped and depressed—instead of with shoulders correctly squared and lower back correctly straight! Tell your partner to place a flat free–weight plate on your back if you want more push–up weight.

Stupidly permitting some uncouth thug forcing upon any student his self–styled "shit-load" of detrimental and potentially hurtful repetitions should duly anger and "piss off" anybody! It should indeed rankle conscientious clients enough to strive to put such fitness shysters out of business permanently!

An inane print advertisement for the "National Personal Training Institute," so–called, picturing some grotesquely grimacing guy, shirtless, pretending to be in the midst of performing a strained and strenuous barbell biceps curl, epitomizes the lame-brained pain concept with the caption: "Every-time A Student Screams An Instructor Gets His Wings."

Yeah, well, if any idiot "instructor" ever attempts to compel you to perform any exercise to the extreme point of hurtful pain then by all means do send him flying—with or without his wings!

THREE:

TRAINING TIPS FOR SELECT EXERCISES

"I believe the reason that most people torque their bodies so much is simply to use more weight and show off at the gym— but this should never be your objective if building a classic physique is your goal. They would get more benefits—that is, more results in a shorter period of time— if they simply forgot about the weight and concentrated on doing the movement correctly."—Steve Reeves

TYPICAL TRAINING MISTAKES TO REMEDY

This section isn't meant at all to repeat or rehash Steve's training or workout "schedule" as he preferred to call it rather than refer to it as a repetitive routine. Obtain Steve's bodybuilding book to learn and master the complete practice of real championship bodybuilding. Instead, this section intends only to point out some of the most redundantly observed but most readily remedied training pitfalls.

Deltoids(Shoulders)
Upright Rowing(barbell)

Grip the barbell in the middle with your hands only chin–width apart with your thumbs–in. Keep your elbows out as you lift the barbell slowly and smoothly to your chin. Flex and lock your lat(back) muscles throughout this movement to target your front deltoids(shoulders)by disengaging your trapezius muscles from doing the work. Don't drop the weight during the negative(eccentric)part of the movement. Don't pause at the bottom part of the negative movement. Pause instead at the top of the positive(concentric)part of the movement. The same goes for performing the standing–front–barbell–raise for the front deltoids: stand with your back straight hanging the barbell at arms' length with a close grip against your upper thighs. Raise the bar straight out and up until it's just above your shoulder height. *LIFT* the weight. ***DO NOT WASTE YOUR TIME AND EFFORT SWINGING UP THE WEIGHT FOR MOMENTUM***. Pause. Return slowly to the starting position while lowering the barbell keeping your elbows locked throughout the movement.

Seated Press(dumbbells)

If you're going to perform seated, simultaneous, palms–forward, thumbs–in dumbbell presses for the side shoulders then don't waste your time and effort by doing those half–arse movements. Start your presses in the fully contracted position level with your shoulders which you intend to target. Complete your presses in the fully extended, topmost position overhead, pausing for a beat before lowering the weight slowly and smoothly to a point level with your shoulders again. If you're lowering the dumbbells only halfway down to handle heavier weight then get over it, reduce your poundage and do it correctly—or just don't do it at all! You might best benefit by performing instead seated Alternate Press(dumbbells)—lifting one weight at a time, palms–in, while alternately switching sides throughout the set.

Bent–Over Lateral Raises(dumbbells)

Don't bend over in a half–arse position with bent elbows using your arm and back muscles to generate momentum by swinging the dumbbells upwards like some do–do bird trying to take flight! Bend forward at the waist until your torso is at a 90–degree right angle to your legs. Keep your arms perfectly straight and lift the dumbbells laterally—up and out to the sides—until parallel with your shoulders. Pause in the fully contracted position before lowering the dumbbells slowly and smoothly, keeping your arms straight. You might best benefit by performing this movement face–down(prone)upon either a high flat bench or a high incline bench to avoid any stress to your lower back. You can also perform this movement while standing bent–over with your forehead resting against the back of a seat or some other waist–level upright object. The same goes for doing standing–side–lateral–raises grasping your dumbbells at arm's length, palms–in, against your upper thighs: ***DO NOT WASTE YOUR TIME AND EFFORT SWINGING UP THE WEIGHTS FOR MOMENTUM.*** Slowly raise the dumbbells to a position just above shoulder height, pausing before slowly returning to the starting position keeping your arms straight throughout the movement.

Pectorals(Chest)
Supine Bench Press(barbell)

Keep a medium wide grip on the barbell to maintain a steady and even degree of demand on the chest muscles from beginning to end of the movement. Grip the bar too close and your press will start easy but finish hard. Grip the bar too wide and your press will start hard but finish easy. Keep your feet flat on the floor throughout the movement. Never arch your back off the bench or drop and bounce the bar off your chest.

Supine Flying Motion(dumbbells)

Today, strict dumbbell flyes are incorrectly confused with dumbbell laterals. Doing dumbbell flyes: hold your dumbbells with an offset grip—meaning you press your thumbs against the inside of the plate and let the rest of the dumbbells hang down against your forearms to sustain the tension on your chest muscles throughout the movement. Start the movement with your arms fully extended overhead in a thumbs–in position. Keep your arms slightly bent at the elbows throughout the entire movement from full extension to full contraction. Lower the dumbbells a little below the bench during the negative(eccentric)part of the movement for a comfortable stretch without hyper–extending your arms. Doing dumbbell laterals: keep your grip in a palms–in position, keep your arms as straight as possible throughout the movement but likewise lower the dumbbells a little below the bench during the negative(eccentric)part of the movement.

Parallel Bar Dip(parallel bars)

Bulk–builders perform this exercise incorrectly the most consistently with frenetic, half–arse movements, bouncing up and down on their bent, flared–out elbows for momentum—either to evade the embarrassment of being powerless to properly press their own bodyweight or to make a deceptive display of strength by dangling an over–heavy dumbbell from their crossed feet throughout their mock movement. To correctly focus on your lower chest muscles: press yourself up to complete extension, locking your elbows close to your sides. Lower yourself as far as you can comfortably to complete contraction, bending your arms, preferably until your armpits are level with your grip on the parallel bars or until your biceps and forearms touch. Do it right, or don't do it!

Supine Pullover for Chest and Ribcage(barbell or dumbbell)

Bulk–builders perform this exercise not only illogically but detrimentally with a downright ludicrous and awkward body position, hanging their lower back down completely off the bench with their shoulder blades pressed against the bench and their bent knees supporting their askew body weight. Why stress at once both your knees and lower back so senselessly? A potent dose of common sense is in order here. Lie back on the bench lengthwise as it was made for. Keep your arms straight throughout the movement from start(pressed fully extended overhead)to finish(lowered down and back fully extended until the weight is level with the bench). When working with a barbell rather than a dumbbell keep your grip shoulder–width apart with thumbs–in. If you must tempt fortune at making a splashy display then at least do it correctly: lie across the bench with your upper back completely supporting your torso by hanging your head down off the side of the bench, keeping your body and legs almost straight to avoid stressing your knees and lower back while dropping your hips to raise your rib cage. Perform your pullovers with your body in this correct—and safe(and commonsensical)—position!

Lats(Back)
One-Arm Row(dumbbell)

Bulk–builders perform this exercise incorrectly with frenetic movements by jerking the weight up and down to and from their chest and torque–ing their torsos—once more to make mock displays of strength. Never lift the weight to your chest. Never lift the weight any higher than your hip—inside of which should be the dumbbell's contracted destination—keeping your weight under control throughout the movement in either direction.

Low-Pulley Lat Row(seated cable row)

Bulk–builders perform this exercise incorrectly by jerking and heaving their whole bodies back and forth in a preposterous seesaw movement for momentum—once more to make mock displays of strength. Keep your upper body bent slightly forward at your waist with your shoulders back throughout the movement. Lean forward and move your arms only back and forth in a controlled manner with full extension and full contraction. Pull the low–pulley handles to your waist—not to your chest. Target your lats by working your lats—not your lower back! Pull the weight to your chest only when doing bent–over rows with a barbell. The same goes for performing the standard bent–over–long–bar–rowing movement: straddle the bar with your knees slightly bent, bending forward until your torso is parallel to the floor, holding the bar right behind the plates with one or both hands. Pull the bar straight up until the plates touch your chest, keeping your elbows in close. ***DO NOT WASTE YOUR TIME AND EFFORT BY JERKING UP THE WEIGHT FOR MOMENTUM***. Pause. Return to the starting position by slowly lowering the bar without letting the plates touch the floor.

Biceps(Arms)

Always work your biceps after your lats and before your triceps. Your just completed lat work thoroughly warms up your arms for working your biceps. Working your triceps before your biceps tightens the skin on your upper arm and makes getting peak contractions from doing biceps curls unduly difficult.

Standing Curl(barbell)

Bulk–builders perform this exercise awkwardly, jerking the weight up and down with their elbows flared out like clucking chickens while swinging their upper bodies back and forth in a seesawing motion for momentum—once more to make mock displays of strength. Keep your elbows pressed in tight against your sides. Never flare out your elbows. Never raise your elbows forward for leverage—keep your elbows straight and vertical. Strictly curl and lower the weight in a controlled manner throughout the movement. Doing otherwise uselessly stresses your elbow joints. Notice how skinny guys aping bulk–builders plop themselves down onto benches while groping their stressed elbows in pain after performing this movement so hurtfully!

Preacher Curl(barbell)

Bulk–builders perform this exercise incorrectly by jerking the weight up and down with flared–out elbows and half–arse movements while leaning with their upper back and shoulders for leverage—once more to make mock displays of strength. Adjust the cushion to fit flush and tight beneath your armpits. Never flare out your elbows, keeping them aligned at shoulder–width with your upper arms kept close–in. Curl the weight in a controlled manner with complete contraction (until your biceps and forearms touch)and complete extension.

Alternate Curl(dumbbells)

Bulk–builders perform this exercise incorrectly by alternately bouncing and swinging up one dumbbell in one hand from their hip while dropping down the second dumbbell in the other—typically with their el-bows flared out to make mock displays of strength. Offset your grip by holding each dumbbell with your little finger pressed against the upper plate while let-ting the rest of the dumbbell hang down. Keep your elbows pressed tight against your sides. Alternately curl the weights in a controlled manner, moving only the forearms with complete contraction and complete extension while keeping your upper arms completely motionless or stationary. That same strict style ap-plies equally to seated concentration curls and simul-taneous dumbbell curls.

Triceps(Arms)
Triceps Press–down(high pulley bar, standing or kneeling)

In spite of how consistently you might see bulk–builders performing this exercise incorrectly it's **NOT**, I must stress, a frenetic triceps *JERK*–down exercise! Space your grip narrowly on the bar only a hand–width apart. Keep your elbows pressed tight against your sides without letting your elbows rise with the weight during the contraction or negative(eccentric)

part of the movement. Contract and extend completely in a controlled manner, moving only your forearms
while keeping your upper arms completely motionless
or stationary.

French Press–Behind–Neck(dumbbell)

Bulk–builders perform this exercise with half–
arse movements by failing to fully lower their forearms and so falling short of complete contraction—
once more to make mock displays of strength. Position
your elbows right next to your ears and keep them
there. Contract and extend completely in a controlled
manner, moving only your forearms while keeping
your upper arms completely motionless or stationary. Lower the dumbbell behind your head as far as
your elbow joints will permit to get the utmost stretch
and to achieve the fullest possible range of motion.
The same goes for doing a one–arm–triceps–extension–behind–your–neck with a dumbbell, alternating
arms: lower the weight behind your head while keeping your upper arm upright throughout but without
moving your elbow until your biceps and forearm
touch.

Bent-Over Triceps Extension(dumbbells)

In spite of how consistently you might see bulk–
builders performing this exercise incorrectly it's
NOT, I must stress, a frenetic triceps **JERK**–back-
and–up extension! Grip a dumbbell in each hand to
do simultaneous extensions for best benefit. Stand
bent at the waist(at least 90 degrees)with your feet
shoulder–width apart. Rest your head on a high seat
or roughly equivalent spot against some flat upright
surface. Align your upper arms parallel to your sides.
Hold in your elbows close. Extend the dumbbells si-
multaneously in a controlled manner back and up,
moving only your forearms while keeping your upper

arms completely motionless or stationary. Pause with the weights at the top of the movement. *Resist* the weights as you contract slowly to the starting position. Of course you can also perform this movement by alternating arms one at a time.

Legs
Lunge–in–Place(dumbbells)

Contemporary bulk–builders and self–styled trainers alike so incorrectly practice and instruct this particular leg exercise as to make it an unduly painful *KILLER* to the knees and knee joints. Hold a dumbbell palms–in in each hand with your arms at your sides. Keep your back perfectly straight. Step forward with one leg a lengthy *TWO* feet or so—this is *NOT* a *SHORT*, half–arse step! Bend your knee slightly past your big toe until your thigh is parallel to the floor. Keep your opposite leg as *STRAIGHT* and as comfortably *STRETCHED* as possible. *DO NOT* stress the knee of your opposite leg by dropping it down to the floor as so typically and so *HURTFUL-LY* mis–taught today. Pause. Return to the standing position. Repeat with your other leg.

Leg Curl/Leg Extension(Machines)

Work your hamstrings(back thighs)before working your quadriceps(front thighs)only when using leg machines. Work your hamstrings by doing leg curls on machines afterwards when you're doing free–weight squats for your leg work. If you work your quadriceps first you won't be able to do your squats as well or lift as much weight. Perform your leg curls and extensions on machines in a controlled manner with complete contractions and complete extensions. Watch the weight plates and concentrate on letting them almost touch during the negative(eccentric)part of the movement.

Calf Raises(leg–press machine)

Bulk–builders likewise perform this exercise quite incorrectly by uselessly bouncing the weight up and down on the balls of their feet with half–arse movements—once more finally to make mock displays of strength! Position your shoulders under the machine's parallel extensions. Stand with your feet roughly a foot apart. Keep your back straight and your legs locked. Raise up as high as possible on the balls of your feet. Pause. Lower your heels as low as possible to get the utmost stretch. Return to starting position. Always strive for a full range of motion. Always raise all the way up and lower all the way down in strict style. Keep your toes pointed straight ahead and concentrate on putting most of your weight on your big toes as you go up and down in a controlled manner.

Back
Forward Bend/Good Morning(barbell, seated or standing)

This fantastic lower back exercise is preferably performed seated and is superior to dead–lifts for the very same reason: your glute muscles kick in to do the work when you do dead–lifts or perform the forward bend standing. Rest a barbell behind your neck on your trapezius muscle while seated. Hold the bar with a wide thumbs–in grip. Bend far forward at the waist in a controlled manner until your torso is parallel to the floor. Pause. Return to the starting position. If you suffer lower back pain or sciatica this is the number one exercise which will offer you the utmost stretch and most permanent therapeutic relief. After all, Steve reminded us, "those muscles are the greatest protection in the world for the spine."(***Dynamic Muscle Building***, Page 73).

Midsection(Abdominals/Obliques)

No, admittedly I don't have photo–shopped alligator abs—but nor do I believe having them is at all desirable. Personally I've never wanted to look like an oversized lizard creature that walked upright on two legs! Most athletes tend either to over–train or under–train their midsections. Maintaining a flat and firm midsection strikes a proper balance. If you strive to look sickly and skinny like self–styled "fitness celebrity/personality," John Basedow, then almost anyone can attain alligator abs if they starve themselves and lose their subcutaneous fat tissue to such a startling—and unhealthy—degree. Weighing in at only about 200 pounds at 6'3" Basedow is more or less 30 pounds underweight by classic physique standards, presuming he has medium–sized bones. In fact he looks more like a skeletal model for the artistic reference book, *Gray's Anatomy*, than a fitness model! Or a Holocaust victim with moderate muscular development! Still, he's an estimable entrepreneur and a better fitness model to emulate than any unfit and unhealthy bulk–builder. So I mention him only by way of physique–comparison.

Abdominals make up a support structure which sustains the internal organs and empowers the muscles of the lower back, hips and thighs to function effectively. Feeble or undeveloped abdominals frequently cause chronic back pain. So strengthen and trim your midsection with the exercise which most closely mirrors the natural function of the muscle group—the abdominals—being worked:

Crunches(correct)

Lie supine on a flat surface. Bend your legs to the floor at a 90–degree angle. Place your palms on your **FOREHEAD(DO NOT** clasp your hands behind your head to stress your neck and prevent your abdominals from properly performing their contractions!). Keep your lower back on the flat surface at all times. Point your elbows toward your knees. Exhale as you curl your upper body forward and upward to the point of complete abdominal contraction with your elbows touching your knees—or as close as possible to that position. *HOLD* the crunch in that position for a strict *TWO* count without cheating yourself of that utmost, concentrated contraction. Inhale as you slowly and smoothly return your upper body to the starting position. Repeat until you can no longer maintain strict style—taking in your breath on your way down, letting out your breath on your way up.

This is one exercise you can perform anytime almost anywhere—even in front of your television set—so there's absolutely no excuse for neglecting to do it. For some cheap sexist entertainment I'll do a whole half hour's worth of correct crunching during the *Girls Gone Wild* infomercial! So do whatever it takes to make it fun and get you through it. I've done opportunistic crunching even on public cement benches while waiting for rides or trains. If nothing else the conspicuous reactions of innocent bystanders can prove to be quite diverting!

Bent–Knee Curl–Up(bodyweight)

Lie supine on the floor with your legs bent and your calves resting on a low flat bench. Place your palms upon your forehead. Curl forward and upward until your elbows touch your knees or as far as you can. Pause. *DO NOT WASTE YOUR TIME AND EFFORT JERKING UP YOUR UPPER BODY FOR MOMENTUM*. Return to the starting position. The same goes for doing sit–ups lying on the floor with your legs raised, knees slightly bent, and your feet against a wall: *DO NOT WASTE YOUR TIME*

68

AND EFFORT JERKING UP YOUR UPPER BODY FOR MOMENTUM. Sit up as far as possible. Pause. Return to starting position. Simple.

Knee–Up(vertical station)

Position your forearms on the armrests. Brace your back against the backboard and grip the handles. Raise up your knees to parallel level, bending your legs. Pause in that knee–contracted position and hold for a beat. Straighten and lower your legs to their starting position *WITHOUT WASTING YOUR TIME AND EFFORT BY SWINGING YOUR LEGS UP AND DOWN FOR MOMENTUM.* The same goes for doing straight–leg raises at the waist. Forget swinging—it gets your midsection *NOTHING*.

To reiterate: *HOW* you execute your exercises and perform your movements is eminently more important than what exercise you do or what weight you lift!

FOUR:

HOW TO WEIGHT–TRAIN CORRECTLY (IN STEVE'S OWN WORDS TO THE MASS MEDIA)

"Never really known as a gym rat, Steve's personal philosophy was to train hard, then forget training and be a normal person who happened to have the adjunct of muscle. Nearly 50 years after he last competed, Steve Reeves is a bodybuilding icon whose physique is always presented as 'Exhibit A' in any bodybuilding debate concerning aesthetics versus mass."—International Federation of Bodybuilding Hall(IFBB)of Fame

Training Order and Exercises
(*Muscle & Fitness*, May 1983)

•"I always liked to work my shoulders first, doing upright rowing, presses–behind–neck and dumbbell lateral raises. I worked chest next, doing very wide–grip bench presses, incline presses with dumbbells and flyes. Next, for my lats I did chins–behind–neck, seated pulley rowing and decline pullovers. For biceps I did only incline dumbbell curls with a rear stop bar to prevent cheating. I did ten sets of 5 reps, starting with 75–lb. dumbbells, and never going below 50 lbs. or resting between sets. Next, I did triceps extensions on the overhead pulley, then on the flat bench with a barbell, and one–arm triceps extensions on the bench using a dumbbell and crossing over to the opposite shoulder. For thighs I did parallel squats with 400 lbs., followed by four sets of front squats with lighter weight, 10–12 reps each exercise. Seated good mornings, leg curls and calf raises completed the program. For upper body I did three sets on each exercise, a total of nine sets each body–part, generally 7–11 reps. I don't believe a body–part needs more than that if a person really concentrates on the muscle being worked and trains with a super high intensity."(Page 132).

Total Body Training
(*Muscle & Fitness*, May 1983)

•"I trained three times a week, two hours each workout. If I had worked my calves and waist more, which I didn't need, I would have had to use the split system. I preferred to train my entire body each workout, three days a week, and rest four days. That's not many training days, but I trained with such high intensity that my rest days seemed like mere pauses."(Page 133).

Train With Concentration
(*Muscle & Fitness*, May 1983)

•"The mind is everything. I used to train with such concentration I would get furious if anyone interrupted with attempted conversation. My workout partner would come to my rescue and tell people not to bother me, that I'd be happy to answer their questions when I finished my workout."(Page 134).

Train With Strict Style
(*Muscle & Fitness*, May 1983)

•"I like to handle as much weight as I can with good style. I don't try to make the weight heavier than it is by doing extremely slow movements, or lighter than it is by using fast swinging or bouncing movements."(Page 134).

Training The Chest
(*Flex*, February 1993)

•"I liked to do my bench presses with a wide grip, my incline dumbbell presses with a slight rotation of the palms and my dumbbell flyes with an offset grip. With wide–grip bench presses, if your grip was too close, you had a slow start and fast finish. If your grip was too wide, you had a fast start and slow finish. However, if your grip was wide, but not too wide, the resistance was perfectly proportionate all the way through the range of motion. As for incline dumbbell presses, I'd go up to 110 pounds, but use really good style. I would have my palms face forward at the beginning of the movement, when the dumbbells were on my chest, and then slowly rotate them inward as I lifted the 'bells until they faced each other and the weights touched at the very top of the movement. The flye motion with an offset grip was performed by extending my arms above my chest as one would for a normal flye, except my palms would be facing the wall in front of me. My grip was offset in that my thumb and index finger were jammed against the plates at one end of the dumbbell, so that the remainder or lower part of the dumbbell was hanging down toward the ground. This offset grip provided more resistance throughout a greater range of motion. Dumbbell flyes typically are like bench presses with a close grip; they start out difficult and then get progressively easier toward the top or finish of the movement. This means an imbalance in resistance, but when flyes are performed my way, with the thumbs in, toward each other, the resistance is constant and difficult all the way up and all the way down."(Pages 37-38).

Train With Extreme Concentration
(*All Natural Muscular Development*, November 1997, Volume 34, Number 11)
•"I've always been into extreme concentration. Whenever I work out, I concentrate exclusively on the muscle I'm training. When I was competing for Mr. America, I'd concentrate on every bodybuilding exercise I performed, doing them nice and slow so that I could really feel the movement all the way up and all the way down. I've always used a full range of motion and it really worked out well for me. What you have

to establish is a superior line of communication between your brain and your muscles. And you can only do that two ways: by concentrating and by practicing muscle–control exercises in your spare time when you're not working out. Muscle control exercises are when you can flip or twitch your muscles at will; that is, getting them to flex or twitch through brief, voluntary contractions. When you can do this, then you have established a solid line of communication between your mind and your muscles. By building up a greater, superior line of communication between my brain and my muscles, I was able to develop much faster and easier than most of my contemporaries."(Page 148).

Rest and Recuperation Between Workouts
(*All Natural Muscular Development*, November 1997, Volume 34, Number 11)

•*Rest* "is just as important as the workout itself in building muscle size. A lot of bodybuilders don't have adequate recuperation in between their workouts. They work out, then they work out, and then they work out again—they're tearing down muscle and not giving it enough rest for optimum growth...You have to remember that working out is a tearing down of tissue that has to be rebuilt. And if you train too hard and don't get enough rest, you're not going to make progress. Some people make progress in three months that others can't in a year because the other people just work too hard and don't get enough rest. Don't be one of those people. Train hard, but get adequate rest and recuperation in between workouts—and you'll grow progressively bigger muscles that are fully shaped and impressive to look at 365 days of the year."(Page 148).

Train Your Small Muscles First, Large Muscles Last

(*All Natural Muscular Development*, January 1998, Volume 35, Number 1)

•"Many people start their training by working the legs first; the theory being that larger muscles should be worked first because they take more energy to work than smaller muscles. Besides, if a bodybuilder would work the smaller muscles first, he/she wouldn't have enough energy to work the bigger muscles later in the workout. I don't agree. I believe that the legs should be worked near the end of your workout, after you've worked the major muscles of the upper body. Here's why: Because your legs are the largest and strongest muscles in the body, they are needed to form a strong foundation of support while you are doing most exercises for the upper body. Without this strong foundation, you won't be able to put out the maximum effort while working the smaller muscles of the upper body. I also believe it is better for your body to warm up and increase the circulation gradually by doing exercises that don't put too much demand on your system too quickly. By working the smaller muscles first, then working legs near the end of your training, you accomplish this. Approximately 80% of your blood is located in your legs and glutes(which are worked while you exercise the other body areas). So, if you work your legs first, you will be bringing even more blood down into the lower extremities, thus drawing it away from the smaller muscles in your upper body. All of this makes for an unnecessary and undesirable demand on your system(forcing the body to pump large amounts of blood against gravity), once you start making the body bring the blood back to the upper body when you begin working the smaller muscles. The bottom line is: If you want the best results from your workouts, start with the smaller muscles of the upper body and work down to your legs."(Page 132).

Tips To Train For A Natural, Classic, Proportionate and Symmetrical Physique

(*All Natural Muscular Development*, February 1998, Volume 35, Number 2)

•Complete Extension and Complete Contraction. "You must exercise your muscles through their fullest possible range of motion. This means complete extension and complete contraction in perfect style—but get every last rep you can from every set you perform."(Page 128).

•Train Wide To Be Wide. "It's always been my belief that if you think wide and train wide, you'll become wide. That's why I do a lot of wide–grip exercises—like wide–grip bench presses, wide–grip chins behind neck, press–behind–neck with a wide–grip and so on."(Page 128).

"I was amazed at the brevity of his workout and the obvious results he obtained," Fred Fornicola wrote for *NaturalStrength.com*, summarizing Steve's training schedule. "He trained full-body workouts with 1–2 sets per movement using mainly multi–jointed exercises to failure three times a week. I remember this very well because there were pictures of him on the beach with all these beautiful women hanging all over him while he commented how others languished in the gym about their training. Now I know the man had good, no make that great genetics, but he had the right idea training briefly, infrequently and intensely to facilitate progress in his bodybuilding endeavor."

I've observed far too many people, especially those misguided groupies of some amateur bulk–builder, doing just that—languishing in gyms. They'll work out hour after hour, day after day, day in and day out, month after month, but extremely lackadaisical, posing in the mirrors, looking repeatedly and hoping against hope for expected developments in their physiques which simply never, ever appear. Sad. Don't be one of them! Train Steve's way and you won't be: short, sweet but intense!

"Instead," Steve advised, "use your brain and train wisely, in the most efficient manner possible."(*Dynamic Muscle Building*, Page 121).

FIVE:

PRACTICAL (NOT PERRICONE) PRESCRIPTION FOR YOUTH

"A person's health and performance capacity depend predominantly on him going considerably beyond the normal resting figures for respiration, thereby increasing oxygen–supplying capacity."—
Steve Reeves

"Hey, I'm 42!" spouts a nameless but wisely long since un–featured "fitness model" for the so–called "Bowflex" commercial. "And I'm in better shape now than when I was 22!"

Well, maybe. At least this guy displays some modest musculature but by his excessively weathered and worn face he scarcely qualifies as a poster child for youth! In fact, he looks 52 if he's a day—and if you've ever seen his short spot on television you know exactly who I'm talking about!

Body by Jake's infomercial for the so–called "Total Body Trainer" and its associated "Simple Seven" circuit workout likewise briefly features "Big Wave Surfer," Ken Bradshaw, who supposedly at my age or "almost 50"—or so Jake gushes—"is in better shape than most 20–year–olds!"

Well, again, maybe. By his fairly lean physique, perhaps, but scarcely by his coarse and craggy face!

To put it quite bluntly: in both cases these two guys by their battered faces look their ages or like they're aging fast. In a word: *old!*

As with most of today's contemporary "fitness" gurus—like 50–plus pilates "guru," Mari Winsor—their typically timeworn faces with their baggy eyes and saggy necks betray their real ages despite their sometimes lean or muscular physiques. But the real point of this section is: you can retain and maintain at any age a face which looks as youthful and vital as your physique by following a simple and practical prescription which costs little but pays off big–time in the way of true health and fitness benefit! "Just remember," Steve reminded us, "a man can weigh 175 pounds and look good or bad. It's primarily a matter of conditioning. It isn't how much you weigh. It is the quality of your body."

TIPS FOR MAINTAINING TRUE YOUTH AND VITALITY

•**Aerobics Exercise**. Oxygen consumption is what really empowers and energizes our bodily engines to be physically active and to function physically to our utmost capacity. And only by physical exertion can we fully inspire—or take in—ten times as much oxygen through our lungs than when we sleep. In a trained athlete oxygen intake can be increased 20 times the amount(five liters)of the quarter–liter per minute consumed at rest. All told, it's quite enough to consistently practice a tenfold intake of oxygen consumption for lengthy time periods. So the more efficiently we breathe and respire the more oxygen we transport to the bloodstream and the greater amount of *epinephrine* gets absorbed and utilized by our system. *Epinephrine* is a hormone and natural stimulant secreted by the adrenal gland which naturally invigorates you, making you feel more alive and vital. Practically speaking, in terms of training that translates into regular and vigorous aerobics exercise in the form of cycling, running, swimming or walking for a minimum of three to five days per week for a minimum of 20 to 30 minutes per session depending on your aerobics capacity and physical ability. If you do nothing else to keep fit, hale and hearty, consistent and frequent aerobics exercise is the best and most effective activity to engage in and the most beneficial and valuable investment you can ever make in your overall health and longevity. "I believe in running," Steve confided in his bodybuilding book's bodybuilding seminar. "In fact, I used to run the mile just for exercise years ago and I always tried to complete it within five minutes. I used to do that about twice a week. The world record wasn't even four minutes at that time. I worked up to that, too. I paced myself." Or when Steve once lived in Switzerland he'd hike for two to three hours a day! "In Europe," *Muscle & Fitness* magazine reported, "Steve was running regularly long before jogging became popular in America. During one six–month period he ran the mile at least four times a week, every time in under five minutes. He believes in the ground–gaining action of running as opposed to jogging, and not more than three miles for maximum benefit. In Europe, he came to depend much on running to keep in shape."(May 1983, Page 186). "I believe in running," Steve reiterated. "In fact, I used to run the mile just for exercise years ago, and I always used to try to be within five minutes or five minutes and a few seconds. I used to do that about twice a week and try to get within five minutes each time."(***Dynamic Muscle Building***, Page 17). As for myself, at past 50 I normally run on the treadmill at least two to three miles at a pace of 8.0—or the equivalent of 7.5–minute miles—though my pace may range anywhere from 7.0 to 7.5 to 8.0 to 8.5 depending upon my current state of conditioning. I've been known to do five minute warm–up runs at 9.0. To demonstrate their complete lack of aerobic capacity I'd challenge any bulk–builder who was just ten pounds over their classic physique weight for their height and bone structure—even if they were ten, twenty or even thirty years my junior—to try and keep up with me! Any takers? If you're a real bodybuilder and can keep up(surpass me, all the better!) then don't get smug and self–satisfied—I'll happily compliment and congratulate you! I'm not out to outdo anybody, as it were; I'm out only to advocate and advance total(not half–arse)fitness, health and vitality. Just as there are half–baked, half–arse exercise movements in bodybuilding training there are half–baked, half–arse bulk–builders who carelessly neglect their aerobic conditioning to their long–term fitness and health detriment. They're just cosmetic bulk–builders whose bulk is but skin–deep. Don't be one of them! *Be a bodybuilder fitted for functional performance as well as mere form*. Whether you do your aerobic conditioning before or after your weight training is strictly a matter of personal preference. I prefer before since it energizes and thoroughly warms up my muscles even though fatigue obliges me to lift lighter poundage than after when fatigue would oblige me to run less energetically with less intensity. So forget altogether that extremely limited and redundantly repeated "cardio" concept. There's cardio–vascular(related to the blood and circulation), then there's cardio–pulmonary(related to the lungs). So saying you're doing "cardio" doesn't distinguish between which thing you're talking about, or both. Aerobic, on the other hand, means "with oxygen," and so necessarily includes both your heart and circulatory and pulmonary systems. Devoutly do your *aerobics* exercise to beneficially increase not only your heart–rate but also your oxygen–intake capacity!

•**Power–Walking**. Sports combining aerobic and anaerobic conditioning to a fairly balanced degree—building muscular endurance, muscular strength and a high degree of aerobic capacity—are cross–country skiing, distance rowing and distance swimming. Seasonal weather along with the absence of natural or human–made amenities like lakes, mountains, rivers or Olympic–sized swimming pools can pose formidable obstacles to the practice of such sports. A most effective alternative to these sports is Steve's innovative, low–impact variation of **POWER–WALKING** erect with progressive resistance, which he originated long before it ever became fashionable. Power–walking is a more strenuous version of brisk walking whereby you breathe rhythmically while lengthening your stride and vigorously swinging your arms pendulum–style in opposition to your leg movements, thereby working all your major muscle groups. And as a rule, the more muscle groups worked during exercise—especially the larger muscles below your belt which make up 75 to 80 percent of your total muscle mass—the more calories or energy you expend. Incidentally, that's why you should avoid resorting to ski–or–step machines which tempt you to grab or grip a crossbar or handles thereby considerably reducing your resistance—unless of course you aspire simply to emphasize building upper body strength at the expense of your aerobic benefit; and if you feel you must utilize such machines then release and completely let go of the crossbar or handles so that you can make the most of the machine by making the most of moving more muscle groups! Begin then by lengthening your power–walking stride. Once you perfect a lengthened stride—walking heel–to–toe with your knees slightly bent and driving your legs with your glutes(or hip muscles)—change your cadence by power–walking faster. Vigorously swinging your arms by your sides up to at least shoulder–height(45 degrees)and back past your hips(30 degrees)—palms–in facing each other—will acclimate you to power–walking quicker with your longest possible stride. Drive forward with your butt—not your toes. Focus on breathing rhythmically and deeply into your gut—not just into your chest. Later on you can increase your power–walking intensity by going for longer distances, over courses with inclines and carrying additional weight resistance(like ankle, hand and waist weights)while walking. Set an early goal of power–walking a half mile in eight minutes. Gradually work up to power–walking a full mile in 14 minutes(if you're 5–feet–6 or shorter)and 12 minutes(if you're 5–feet–7 or taller). Power–walk 30 minutes a day for four days a week for best benefit. Power–walk two to three miles to get in shape. Power–walk one to two miles to stay in shape. "Power–Walking is an ideal supplemental exercise for the bodybuilder," Steve told *Muscle & Fitness* magazine. "It works on the progressive resistance principle, is performed at a high intensity, creates an aerobic effect, burns fat and provides the detailed muscular cuts every bodybuilder strives for. Power–Walking is also virtually injury–free. It doesn't have the up–and–down, injury–causing jolting motion which you encounter while jogging. When Power–Walking, you take a smooth progression of steps with one foot remaining on the ground at all times."(May 1983, Page 134). "I think Power–Walking would be an ideal aerobic exercise for the bodybuilder because it has been designed with bodybuilding considerations," Steve added. "Bodybuilders are trained to exert maximum effort against resistance. Power–Walking permits this, whereas free running, more a function of speed, doesn't have the same resistance effect."(Page 190). Consult Steve's book—***Power Walking***—to attain complete and correct instruction in power-walking techniques.

•**Treadmill Power–Walking**. If you're accustomed to working out on gym treadmills then treadmill power–walking can work up the very same sweat in 20 minutes that you'd break if you ran the same time at a treadmill speed of 8.0. Set as your goal your top power–walking speed of five miles per hour. That translates to a treadmill speed of 5.0. This speed compels you to stride long and swing your arms pendulum–style in opposition to your legs to avoid flying off the end of the treadmill! If you aspire to work even harder then elevate your treadmill's incline and/ or grab a couple 1 to 5 pound hand–weights from your gym's weight room to hold for resistance while swinging your arms. I prefer the three–pound hand–weights myself. Any heavier than five pounds and you can't swing your arms while power–walking through their full range of motion.

At the Medicare age of 65, even suffering from the painful and incurable condition of peripheral neuropathy in the soles of both feet, I still power–walk on the treadmill for two miles five times per week within a time period between 26–32 minutes, swinging a pair of three–pounder dumbbells, as Steve recommended for a 200–pound man 50 years of age or older!

•**Control and Maintain Your Classic Physique Weight**. Most self–styled fitness "experts" preach combining a nutritious diet with aerobics exercise(whether running, jogging, power–walking or cycling)for weight control without ever mentioning how to correctly go about it for best benefit. Continuous and sustained("steady–state")aerobics exercise is best for cutting body–fat and unwanted weight fast. Target your two–to–three miles distance first. Concern yourself with time and intensity later on. Pace yourself to get through your distance however long it takes at whatever speed it takes. Gradually build up your aerobic endurance over time to complete the distance at whatever time and speed you eventually aspire to. Incorporate interval training into your aerobics exercise while conditioning yourself and build-

ing up your endurance. That simply means alternating faster(more intense)with slower(less intense)
levels of exertion over the course of the session. In
short: speed up or slow down your pace but cover your
distance with continuous and sustained effort for the
full duration. Completing your distance will, in the
end, determine the time and intensity best suited to
your own ability and endurance. Cross train to maintain your desired weight. That simply means cycling,
jogging or power–walking to a distant place to run
or swim and then cycling, jogging or power–walking back. Jogging is generally considered to be running slower than eight minutes per mile(7.5 treadmill speed). Swindlers peddling the Bowflex would
gull you to believe that useless piece of junk is the
equivalent of an aerobic circuit training course with a
series of successive exercise stations. Don't get sucked
in to buying either that worthless contraption or the
fraudulent notion propping it up. Actual circuit training amounts to something like an outdoor *par course*
interspersing jogging, power–walking or running in-
between its scattered exercise stations. You can completely dismiss as deceptive, dishonest and outright
fraudulent as well any worthless contraption claim-
ing the capability of making "spot reductions" of fat
deposits in specific parts of the body—like certain abs
apparatuses falsely do. Spot reductions, so–called,
simply don't exist. Body fat stores get reduced, like it
or not, by systematic aerobics exercise combined with
a balanced and nutritional diet. Nothing less, nothing
more. It's just that simple.

As Steve cautions: *"There is no such thing as spot
reduction. The only thing you can do is to tone up
muscles everywhere through proper diet and exercise.
The loss of fat tends to be uniform all over the body in*

proportion to the amount present in any given spot. Vigorous exercise, such as PowerWalking, combined with a sensible diet, provides the best means of reducing your level of body fat...The weight will come off slowly from all over your body."(*PowerWalking*, 1982).

•**Stretch A Lot**. Stretching prevents bodily injuries and to some degree counteracts aging. As muscle tissue loses its elasticity over time joints and muscles tend to stiffen and tighten up. An inelastic, inflexible body is more prone to suffer aches and pains, muscle and tendon tears and ultimately impaired functioning due to loss of range of motion. A typical manifestation of this is the rounding of the back—or "dowager's hump"—due to forward head posture. Warm up your muscles with five minutes of aerobic exercise which makes you break a sweat before stretching(When I'm up to speed I like to do five minutes on the treadmill at 9.0). The absolute best stretching routine I've ever experienced is that practiced by martial artists belonging to the *Japanese Karate Association(JKA)/ International Shotokan Karate Federation(ISKF)*, though before beginning their training they'll often start stretching without any aerobic warm–up and some of their stretches are both hard on and harmful to the knee joints. So proceed with caution there.

•**Drink Lots of Liquids**. Water makes up roughly 65 to 75 percent of the human body. Our bodily fluids are mostly water, which circulates through our blood, blood vessels(arteries, veins and capillaries)and lymphatic system, transporting oxygen and nutrients to cells and tissues while removing wastes through urine and sweat. Water dissolves vitamins, minerals and other nutrients. Water helps our bodies digest and absorb the foods we eat and eliminate digestive waste. Fluids fill both cells and the spaces separating them to keep tissues healthy. Water maintains that delicate balance between dissolved salts and water inside and outside of cells. Water cushions and lubricates our joints and soft tissues. Water helps regulate body temperature. Hydrate your body then by keeping your urine as clear in color as possible— all the more important the older we get. Personally, I'm not that crazy about drinking the regularly recommended eight to 12 cups needed to replenish the water lost daily through sweat and urine. Like Steve then I favor drinking lots of flavored and flavorful liquids like fruit juices. Carbonated beverages are excellent sources of water too. That doesn't mean drinking alcohol, coffee, sodas loaded with refined sugar or juice substitutes loaded with corn syrup. Alcohol and caffeine in particular increase your urine output and so dehydrate your body, causing it to lose water. Drink only 100 percent fruit juices. Whether apple, blackberry, blueberry, cherry, grape, grapefruit, orange, rasberry or tomato I regularly drink upwards of a half gallon(64 ounces)of fruit juice or more a day as I habitually write late at night. Drinking fruit juices in those amounts flushes not only your face but also your bowels—cleansing and purging your entire system—and more effectively than any unnatural laxative. At Trader Joe's stores I've even found bottled blackberry and blueberry juices in stock. Toast your perennial youth then by drinking lots of healthy and tasty liquids! To quote Steve's widow, Deborah Engelhorn–Reeves–Stewart, concerning what Steve himself drank and the wise cue the rest of us can take: "Mostly he consumed juices and water(lots of water)." "Many people think that drinking juice is a great addition to a weight–loss diet," *SF Weekly* "editor," Lisa Crovo—in her paper's self–styled but misguided "Resolution Handbook '03"—quoted purported "expert" and registered dietician, Mikelle McCoin, as contending. "Unfortunately, juice is a very concentrated source of calories." "Eliminate" fruit juices *Parade* magazine's so–called "All–America Get Fit Program"(2007)panel of "experts" likewise witlessly advised. So much for "experts." Ignore then the ignorant who claim that drinking fruit juices detrimentally raises your blood sugar levels due to the ingestion of fructose or "naturally occurring" fruit sugar. As Steve elucidated: "Fructose is made up of different types of molecules that last longer in your system and therefore don't play havoc with your blood sugar levels, having instead a more moderate 'chain–release' effect."(***Dynamic Muscle Building***, Page 124).

•**Sleep A Lot**. Rest and sleep a lot on a fairly firm bed close to an open window to breathe fresh air while sleeping. "I've found over the years another way to assist your nutrition in the repair and growth of your muscle tissue—it's called a 'muscle nap.'" Steve wrote for *All Natural Muscular Development* magazine. "I've found that if you can take even a half–hour nap during, say, your lunch hour—do it. I've done it all my life. In any kind of work I've been involved in, I've always been given about an hour for lunch, and I'd just lay down on the floor(or wherever I happened to be)and take a half–hour nap. Today, not having to get back to work, I'll take an hour–and–a–half nap. Even when I was making movies, I'd take an hour's nap at lunch time. The bodybuilding dividend is that the sleep gives you complete relaxation of both your body and your mind and, lest we forget, your nervous system, which has also gone through a demanding workout. So, the muscle nap gives your body complete relaxation and, when you're relaxed, your body can mend itself and recover and grow easier."(November 1997, Volume 34, Number 11, Page 148).

•**Make Love A Lot**. Refresh, relax, renew and thoroughly soothe your system to the utmost degree by supplementing your lengthy sleep with lots of lovemaking with your favorite and most faithful companion. If bulk–builders move sluggishly when they merely walk imagine what lumbering lovers they must make! Women of cultivated taste and refined discrimination have no use for bulk–builders and won't give them the time of day anyway! "While I know that many guys admire your physique," Katelyn R. wrote Steve in *All Natural Muscular Development Magazine*, "so do us women! Little do so many of the guys today realize that building such a huge, drug–bloated body has absolutely zero sex appeal to the majority of women. Wake up guys!"(March 1998, Volume 35, Number 3, Page 110).

•**Practice Healthy Hygiene Habits**. My habitual daily routine goes like this: first I brush my teeth and floss with a tarter–control, whitening toothpaste and easy–glide floss(Steve brushed his teeth and massaged his gums regularly with baking soda and salt). Next, I gargle thoroughly with undiluted *Listerine* or its drugstore generic equivalent. I gargle multiple times to cleanse both my mouth and, jutting my jaw far forward and tilting my head way back, my deepest throat. At 50–plus—to the constant and ceaseless amazement of my dentist—I've gotten only two childhood, molar–filled cavities throughout my entire life. Then I thoroughly wash my face and neck with a liberally spread mask of *Noxema* skin cream or its drugstore generic equivalent. Those ancient natural and medicated ingredients like camphor, eucalyptus oil and menthol not only thoroughly cleanse but refresh your face as well. Then I shave, which is so much more bracing after my creamy face–wash. Finally, I take a hot and steamy shower, or bath, after once more covering my face with skin cream, washing my face last to let my face and opened pores benefit most from the shower's steamy vapors. Shampoo before bathing in the shower with a natural shampoo(like *Nature's Gate* biotin, jojoba or keratin), rinsing out your hair last after you've washed the rest of your body. Caring for your face in this specific sequence makes shaving much smoother and totally eliminates the purchase and use of commercial aftershave products! After showering I gently clean my ear canals with cotton swabs dipped in liquid alcohol. Sparingly douse your scalp with a few drops of bottled jojoba oil to make your hair look shiny and youthful which at the same time covers up any light patches of gray. Spouted a dated television commercial for hair cream: "A little dab'll do 'ya!" Try it—you'll like it! Otherwise, if you prefer simply to take a good old–fashioned tub bath then completely plunge yourself and soak in a bathtub full of warm soapy water, which can be equally refreshing and rejuvenating, lathering up both your face with skin cream before shaving and your hair with shampoo before washing and rinsing your scalp.

•**Get Lots of Fresh Air and Sunshine**. Expose your body to the fresh air and sunlight for one to two hours a day whenever weather permits. Limit but don't block your exposure to sunshine—vital to synthesizing your vitamin D. If your skin really required "su–screen" then your body would've been born with it! To promote a blushing and brilliant suntan nutritionally Steve recommended ingesting lots of iron by washing down raisins with lots of carrot juice! "In preparation for the upcoming contests," wrote official biographer, Chris LeClaire, "he incorporated raisins and carrots in his diet, believing that the red in the iron of the raisins and the orange of the carrots worked together to enhance his tan."(Page 70). "I would eat lots of raisins," he says, "and drink enormous amounts of carrot juice. The reason that I did this was that iron in your system makes your skin a little reddish, a blush color, and carrot juice makes you a little orangish. So red and orange together, with a little sun, will give you a real brilliant tan."(Page 111).

•**Practice Face-Friendly Dietary Habits**. Avoid dietary habits detrimental to your facial health and vitality. Don't consume excessive amounts of alcohol, coffee, fat–striated red meat(beef, pork), chips, refined white flour or sugar products(cakes, candy, cookies, crackers, doughnuts, ice cream, pies, sodas) and *DON'T SMOKE OR TAKE DRUGS!* Does anybody really need to mention that? "I've always felt," Steve stressed, "that any unnecessary chemical taken into the body which in any way alters our delicately balanced body chemistry is an insult and a potential danger to our health, longevity and appearance." A positive step you can take is to sweat yourself out often in your gym's steam–heat room if it has one. Humidity helps brace your face!

•**"Put Pep in Your Step and Pride in Your Stride**." That's how Steve advised to walk tall with great posture. We've all observed how many older people tend to chop and shorten the lengthy and springy stride of their youth. Lengthening your stride stretches and strengthens your leg muscles. Longer and limber legs both look and work better. Nowadays, though, you'll see even healthy younger people plodding and trudging along the streets like they're disabled convalescent patients or crippled, decrepit and doddering senior citizens ready for the walking–frame! It would be comical if it weren't so pathetic but if I'd ever walked so sluggishly as a youth among the generation I was reared by I would've gotten a swift butt–kick by one of my elders in the rear! Bulk–builders lumber equally slow and snail–like—just another sensible reason to maintain a body weight proportionate to your height and bone structure!

•**Smile, Don't Scowl!** Nowadays as well you'll see many ostensibly healthy young people not only trudging about but at the same time frowning, glaring, glowering and scowling at passersby for no apparent reason except to look what they misguidedly think to be tough or intimidating to total strangers. Elders in my day would again slap "upside the head" any adolescent–acting spoilt brat who'd moan–and–mope around and sulk to such a childish, self–indulgent degree. Our over–coddled and pampered youth perhaps explains in part why our society suffers today so much rampant violence in our schools. Be that as it may, there's no surer or swifter path to premature aging, bitterness, frustration, menopause and senility than habitual scowling! Scowling makes only lines, wrinkles, animosity, hostility and resentment! Smiling, on the other hand, makes lines perhaps but also good cheer, laughter, pleasantness and serenity! So don't be a scowling, walking, talking joke because the laugh's only on you! If you're really that angry, bitter, tortured, unhappy, wretched or whatever then stop imposing your misery on anyone and everyone in sight and get some emotional or mental *HELP!* At the very least, take a rectifying *ENEMA!* Smile, be happy and stay forever youthful! Your face honestly won't break! *Happiness*, Steve told *Ironman* magazine, "is what makes living an adventure."(February 1999, Volume 58, Number 2, Page 183).

• **Cling To Something From Your Childhood To Stay Child–Like And So Youthful**. For me, it's classic "B" creature features, horror and monster movies and magazines—still the absolute best fun! *FUN* is what those childish, prematurely aging *SCOWLERS* simply don't know how to have and, tragically to their great misfortune, likely never will! *PROFOUNDLY SAD!*

• **Take Life In Healthy Stride**. Don't fanatically obsess or stress–out over anything—fanatical extremism's never worth the time or effort spent on it. So shed any chips from your shoulders and throw away any axes to grind. "You should always try to lead a balanced life," Steve philosophized. "Don't be a fanatic in any way, and always have a positive attitude." As he reiterated to *Flex* magazine: "Don't have too many material demands in life and try to lead a balanced life without being fanatical in any way."(February 1993, Page 113). Or as he told George Helmer in an interview for *Cult Movies* magazine: "First of all, I think to be fit and in shape is a great thing. But it shouldn't dominate and rule your life. I believe your life should be balanced."(Number 18, 1996, Page 43).

• **Conceive To Achieve In Spite of Genetics**. Don't cop out, finally, by constantly falling back upon the negative, nay–saying word: can't! Or by making flimsy alibis and excuses like you don't possess the "genetics" for bodybuilding. True, genetics can and does limit to some degree your ultimate physical development and potential. But you can offset any genetic shortcoming at any age with correct nutrition and training. You can make up for any imbalance in genetics by eating and working out correctly with deep concentration. Depending of course on your natural, God–given body type, Steve suggests that you "create a picture in your mind of how you want your physique to look when you reach your genetic potential." Whenever you have your doubts about your potential development simply recall Steve's practical prescription that "ultimately, you must be your own body architect, your own exterior decorator." He counseled for *All Natural Muscular Development* magazine never to self–impose limitations on your development: "Whenever people try to dissuade you, refuse to listen to them! You can achieve whatever you want to with your bodybuilding…if you want to look like a very well–built human being, then adopt a positive mental attitude and refuse to listen to anyone who tries to discourage you. You should also adopt a similar attitude with regard to your training."(November 1997, Volume 34, Number 11, Page 148). "To maintain," **QUACK** medical director Tim Church, M.D.—and so–called "rising star as an authority on exercise research"—was quoted in a really ridiculous article about the Cooper Aerobics Center in Dallas, Texas(*USA Weekend*, 10–12 January 2003), "you should do it(weight training)once a week. If you want to do it twice a week, that's your priority, but it only really takes once. Why only once a week? Because you're not really going to build up like you did when you were 18 or 20. But once a week will stop the degradation." Well, speak for yourself, Doctor Dumb! I never built myself up or looked even remotely close physique–wise to like I do now when I was 18 or 20(in fact, I was a tall and lanky track runner)! So don't discourage everybody else simply because *YOU DON'T KNOW HOW* to not only "stop the degradation" but also maximally build and develop quality muscle mass *AT ANY AGE!* Disappointingly, even four–time Mr. Universe, Bill Pearl, tried putting a damper on the ardor of "mature"(40–plus)bodybuilders with these unduly discouraging comments made to Gene Mozee of *Graphic Muscle*: "Of course, if you're over forty, you shouldn't set your sights on winning a muscle contest or becoming 'Mr. America' if you are beginning bodybuilding for the first time... But you probably shouldn't train more often than every–other–day when weight training. It takes a great deal of energy to exercise all the major muscle groups with heavy resistance exercise, and if you train daily you might feel a little day–after fatigue that will deplete your reserve strength. Advanced bodybuilders can—you can't." Well, don't let Bill Pearl or anybody else for that matter ever tell you what you "can't" do with your natural classic physique bodybuilding as pioneered and perfected by Steve Reeves. I was already 43 years old when I started training Steve's way so I'm here to correctly attest: I *can!* And so can *you!* It just takes relentless, resolute, steadfast and tenacious *DETERMINATION!* "I'm a man of determination...," Steve confided to *Iron Game History*. "If I set my mind to something. If I don't set my mind to something, I'm just like anybody else...What I figure is that if there's a light at the end of the tunnel and I can see it, no matter how long the tunnel and how dim the light, if I can see it, I'll get there."(December 2000, Volume 6, Number 4, Page 14). No, I won't ever attain the perfect physique of Steve Reeves. Nobody will. Nobody could. But by strong–willed determination I won't ever stop *TRYING* to attain it. Steve's perfect physique is my dim light at the long tunnel's end.

That alone is more than enough to keep me at it! "I honestly believe," Steve assured everybody, "that any boy or man that wants to, can build his body to very good proportions—if he is conscientious and determined to do so. It is strictly a matter of 'stick to it'...anyone who really is serious about building up his body can do so if they have the determination and willpower to do so."(Dynamic Muscle Building, Page 8).

•**Avoid Nagative Naysayers**. Deliberately avoid in your personal and professional associations and relationships those petty people who are chronically critical and cynical, persistently pessimistic and sarcastic or otherwise habitually derisive and disparaging about your natural classic physique training efforts. These envious, resentful and unsupportive individuals, boorish *LOSERS* who thrive on their own extreme immaturity and negativity, seek only to "empower" their own impotence and inadequacies at your expense. Confidently persevere in the certain conviction that you'll definitely develop and excel while these obnoxious *LOSERS* ineptly and ineffectually *FAIL AND STAGNATE*.

§

If the *Blair Witch Project* perpetrated the most outrageous film *HOAX* imaginable upon the moviegoing public since Orson Welles with his reading of H.G. Wells' War of the Worlds gulled thousands of the radio–listening public in 1938 into believing Earth was under attack by invading Martians then Nicholas V. Perricone is presently perpetrating the most outrageous *HEALTH* hoax imaginable upon the health–and–fitness–minded public!

Perricone, a supposed "pioneer in the field of appearance," tours the country foisting upon his gullible public his high–flown "inflammation" theory of aging while peddling his exorbitant and extravagant product line of "Cosmeceuticals," which could more aptly be called fraudulen–ceuticals since the only things there getting inflamed—or more accurately, inflated—are Perricone's pocketbook and suit closet! His website makes clear that he's not attending any "new patients" but quite promptly refers visitors to its "Where to Buy" area. Likewise, his email contact link strictly limits and restricts questions to remain "related to products that Clinical Creations, LLC distributes." And with good and greedy reason: some of his product packages of so–called "topical treatments" can pluck your pocket and cost a pretty Perricone penny—upwards of almost 500 bucks a pop!

This unscrupulous sharper's con game resorts to an age–old come–on: exploit the laziness and vanity of human nature by falsely promising youth through costly emollients, lotions, moisturizers or other counterfeit cosmetics. "What I do have problems with," Steve wrote in a similar vein for *All Natural Muscular Development* magazine, "are people who make money by all the hype they create about their products by feeding off the insecurities of a trusting bodybuilder who's looking for real answers about how to get bigger, stronger, recover faster and have better workouts. This really upsets me. When you see ads making incredible claims or using models that claim they exclusively used that product to get in that condition, it would be wise for you to think twice. I've never seen any supplement—short of a drug—that will produce such miraculous changes in a human body so quickly. None."(December 1997, Volume 34, Number 12, Page 130).

In a CBN News interview Perricone told Pat Robertson what—tragically—too many unsuspecting people want to hear: poor diet is the chief cause of inflammation–inflicted aging and hard work isn't necessary to counteract it.

"But you don't have to work out very hard," Perricone claimed. "You know a walk every day and a few weights is all you need. You don't need to be running marathons, you don't need to be in the gym two hours a day. It's just not necessary. In fact, if you over–exercise, it's pro–inflammatory."

What's "pro–inflammatory" is the extortionate inflation of Perricone's topical products!

Correct diet and nutrition are indeed as necessary to nourishing and nurturing youthful vitality as extreme marathon–ing and power–lifting are unnecessary. But oxygenating your body's cells through constant and consistent aerobic activity—and progressively surpassing certain stages of aerobic capacity and exertion—are all–important and vitally necessary to maintaining and sustaining youthful vitality. And the harder you work at invigorating and vitalizing yourself aerobically the greater your overall fitness and health will benefit.

Any medical doctor who places his high priced "topical" tinctures before aerobics exercise as a youth–promoting, age–resistant counteraction is neither more nor less than an out–and–out *QUACK!* Aerobics exercise is and must remain the first and foremost essential cornerstone supporting any true fitness–and–health strategy!

SIX:
INTELLIGENT NUTRITION AND WEIGHT CONTROL

"The first step required to control your bodyweight begins and ends with what you put into your mouth."—Steve Reeves

Despite the countless deceptive, false and outright fraudulent claims of assorted, self–appointed "fitness experts" and self–styled "fitness gurus" *THERE IS NO MAGICAL MYSTERY OR ESOTERIC "SECRET" TO INTELLIGENT NUTRITION, WEIGHT CONTROL AND KEEPING IN SHAPE!*

Combining accurate knowledge with determined willpower almost anybody can learn how to correctly build muscle, shed body fat and conspicuously change their body shape and size almost at will. That translates more precisely into combining a well–balanced, reduced–calorie diet with regular workouts in a regimen based upon equal portions of exercise, logic, nutrition and self–control. So you most definitely don't need to resort desperately to any fad diets, popping pills or even liposuction to control your weight or reduce your body's fat deposits. Reality and truth are always so absurdly simple: consume excess calories, you gain weight; consume less calories, you lose weight! *PERIOD!*

As Steve put it forthrightly, "You don't need magic pills, newly discovered diets from the geographical social centers of the United States, or Spartan eating habits to control your weight. What will work for you is what worked for me: a program based on equal parts of exercise, proper nutrition, and *common sense...* There is absolutely nothing magical or mystical about winning the battle to lose weight. The key is a rigid adherence to one approach—*COMMON SENSE...* In order to lose weight safely and keep it off permanently, you must do at least two things: eat a nutritionally balanced diet and retrain your eating habits. Above all, your efforts must be guided by *COMMON SENSE...*The keys to 'winning the losing game' are *common sense* and motivation. No magic pills or magic diets will produce the weight loss you are seeking. There is no magic route to follow."(***PowerWalking***, 1982).

Practically speaking, then, your daily diet should distribute itself like this: 60 percent of calories from complex carbohydrates and natural simple carbohydrates(whole fruits), 20 percent of calories from protein and no more than 20 percent of calories from fat. Before your workouts, consume predominantly your complex carbohydrates. "By complex carbohydrates," Steve explained, "I'm referring to foods like grains, legumes and pasta."(***Dynamic Muscle Building***, Page 124). After your workouts, consume protein along with complex carbohydrates throughout the rest of the day to expedite the process of growth and repair for muscle tissue torn down through training. "Again," Steve emphasized, "keep the diet well–balanced with a slight emphasis on your complex carbohydrates, and you'll have abundant energy that will last you not only through the most demanding of workouts, but throughout your normal day–to–day activities as well."

All weight conversion is neither more nor less than the seesaw effect of a weight–control spectrum. At one end are the calories you consume(energy entering your body)while at the other end are the calories you expend(energy exiting your body). If the amount of calories you consume(energy–in)exceeds the amount of calories you expend(energy–out)through exercise and training, you gain weight. If the amount of calories you consume is less than the calories you expend, you lose weight. Maintain your current weight by following a balanced program of diet and exercise which in turn maintains the equilibrium of the weight–control spectrum.

To lose body fat maintain a negative calorie balance by staying more to the energy–out rather than the energy–in side of the weight–control spectrum. Bear in mind the calories of the food and drink you consume on a daily basis relative to the calories you burn through exercise and training. The less body fat you have in proportion to your lean muscle mass the easier it is to lose any leftover unwanted fat since it takes more energy to maintain and sustain muscle than it does fat. "And if you're building muscle," Steve elaborated, "you're building tissue that requires extra calories to fuel—even at rest! This means that, as your muscles get bigger and stronger, they burn more calories just to maintain their existence."(**Dynamic Muscle Building**, Page 124). "An interesting side note in this respect," Steve reiterated, "is that if you can stimulate, say, a pound of lean muscle tissue from a given workout, and you then allow yourself sufficient recovery time to allow from the growth you stimulated to take place, you will have increased your body's rate of metabolism and need of calories—and this means that you are burning more body–fat and becoming lean."(**Dynamic Muscle Building**, Page 120).

§

DISCIPLINE YOUR NUTRITIONAL HABITS
•Eat a balanced diet of healthful and wholesome food.

•Eliminate the intake of fat(saturated, especially), white flour products and refined white sugar products.

•Limit your salt intake. Sodium(salt)is an electrolyte mineral which maintains the balance of our bodily acids and fluids. Specifically it regulates fluid balance by controlling the flow of liquids in and out of every cell. It helps our bodies process and digest carbohydrates and proteins and sparks nerve impulses. It occurs naturally in most foods—even in drinking water. Since it permeates canned, convenience, prepared and processed foods as well as food additives you needn't deliberately add it to your diet—specially since it contributes to high blood pressure in some people.

•Chew completely and slowly. Your blood–sugar level(satiety mechanism)is your body's natural means of letting you know when you've eaten enough. Your food intake prompts your blood–sugar level to respond relatively slow. When you eat too fast you consume more food than you normally would before your satiety mechanism tells you that you're full.

•Eat three regular meals a day.

•Refrain from snacking in–between meals.

•Never eat after six o'clock in the evening.

•Never eat three hours before going to bed.

Knowing and understanding Steve's few simple rules of intelligent nutrition and weight control practices is comparatively easy and effortless. Following those rules frequently proves to be more difficult and demanding. What follows then are some beneficial and helpful nutrition pointers.

Always start your day with a nutritious breakfast or my enhanced and enriched variation on the *"Steve Reeves Power Drink"* or what I call my:

DAILY ENERGY DRINK
(mixed in a blender)

•Banana(1 whole)

•Orange Juice(2–4 cups)

•Strawberries(2–4 by taste/frozen)

•Brewer's Yeast(1 tablespoon/I use *Twinlab SuperRich Yeast Plus*)

•Gelatin/Glucosamine(1 scoop/I use *Knox Nutra Joint Plus Glucosamine*)/Exchangeable with protein powder for those in need of joint restoration and repair. *Bernard Jensen*'s is another great alternate brand of gelatin.

•Wheat Germ(*Kretschmer*)

•Unprocessed Miller's Wheat Bran(fiber fatbuster!)

•Bone Meal Powder(this super–concentrated stuff contains 1300mg of calcium per teaspoon!)

•Bee Pollen Granules(1 tablespoon/whole granules)

•Honey(1 heaping tablespoon/clover)

That sharper, Nicholas V. Perricone, preposterously claims among other things that bananas and honey are "foods to avoid!"

Dubbing the banana the "perfect food," Steve Reeves wrote: "You could also eat as many bananas as you wished throughout the course of the day." Bananas are in fact a chief source of the essential mineral potassium, an electrolyte. Strawberries too are an excellent source of both soluble fiber and vitamin C. And to get his energy up every morning Steve used to pop some bee pollen tablets and drink a tall glass of orange juice with a tablespoon of honey stirred in. That's why I mix bee pollen granules to my daily energy drink—preferable to popping pills!

"The interesting thing about the gelatin," Steve wrote, "is that it's about 87 percent protein but your body can't utilize the protein efficiently because it's missing two key amino acids which you'll find in eggs. So, if you want to do like I did, and use gelatin as the source of your protein, then make sure that you have eggs with it or else it won't work for you...Anyway, you can buy gelatin in any grocery store or health food store. It's about 87 percent protein, as mentioned—but make sure you eat eggs with it or else you won't develop as fast."

Buying inexpensive packets of powdered *Knox* gelatin to mix, refrigerate and store(until it melts and runs)to blend with your daily energy drink is a cheap but cumbersome process. That's why, I suspect, *Knox* today markets its costly but more convenient canister of gelatin—a beneficial source of protein which Steve Reeves farsightedly resorted to in the 1940s!

Alternatively you can substitute a milk–based daily energy drink for an orange juice–based drink, especially if you're trying to gain weight for muscle mass without putting on the fat:

DAILY PROTEIN SHAKE
(mixed in a blender)
- Milk(2 cups/1%-2% milk fat or skim)
- Brewer's Yeast(1 tablespoon)
- Flax(1 tablespoon/milled flaxseed/I use 100% True Gold Milled Golden Flaxseed)
- Protein Powder(2 scoops/tablespoons of soy and/ or egg white)
- Strawberries(2–4/frozen)
- Bee Pollen Granules(1 tablespoon)
- Honey(1 heaping tablespoon)

Steve preferred drinking goat's milk as I do because it's "more complete" than cow's milk. But buying goat's milk sold in supermarkets is costly—unless of course you stock your own goat at home to milk! "I've learned that there is a difference between goat's milk and cow's milk," Steve wrote for *All Natural Muscular Development* magazine. "For one thing, goat's milk is easier to digest and there's a better balance of calcium and phosphorous in goat's milk that you just don't get with cow's milk. And people who are allergic to cow's milk can thrive on goat's milk." Goat's milk, Steve added, "is a superior form of milk. I really think it's fantastic. I drink my goat's milk raw, as raw goat's milk is naturally homogenized because it has such small fat globules that they don't even rise. Plus, as mentioned earlier, it's much easier to digest. It's often perfect for people who are lactose intolerant."(October 1997, Volume 34, Number 10, Page 128).

Generally, the only pill you ever really need to pop with either of these breakfast drinks is a complete multi–vitamin–and–mineral complex though even that may fall short of supplying enough calcium and vitamin D, which is synthesized upon our exposure to sunlight. Preferably you should get your essential and necessary nutrients from eating vitamin–fortified *FOOD*. Never substitute any supplement for eating a healthful, well–balanced, wholesome diet.

"Here's a terrific breakfast:" Steve told *Muscle & Fitness* magazine. "Cut an apple in small cubes, grate a small carrot, add ½ cup of raw oatmeal and the same amount of bran, put in some wheat germ and bee pollen, and pour in milk. I use goat milk. It has it all: roughage, vitamins, minerals, pectin—everything you need. It's a great breakfast."(May 1983, Page 134).

CEREAL/FIBER BREAKFAST
- Bran(1/4 cup)
- Oatmeal(1/4 cup/raw)
- Wheat Germ(1/4 cup)
- Bee Pollen Granules(1 tablespoon)
- Honey(1 heaping tablespoon)
- Milk(goat's)

"Steve is not a timid eater," *Muscle & Fitness*

magazine reported. "Breakfast, for example, is a double helping of goat–cheese omelet and a huge bowl of cereal consisting of raw oats, Grape Nuts, All–Bran, bee pollen, almonds, strawberries and bananas with goat milk, plus a pint of cranberry juice over orange–juice ice cubes."(May 1983, Page 192).

Steve's early "dietary regimen," according to official biographer, Chris LeClaire, consisted of "huge salads, vegetables, fruits of all kinds, a quart of milk a day. A typical breakfast, to Steve's mind the most important meal of the day, was a bowl of wheat cereal with strawberries and cream, four slices of wheat toast with honey on top, three glasses of goat's milk, and four fried eggs. By now(1946)he was emphatic about eliminating any food containing white flour or refined sugar. 'We had a term for it at the gym,' recalls Steve. 'White Death,' meaning refined sugar, devitalized white flour, and salt!' He was insistent about getting nine hours of sleep a night. He drank neither coffee nor tea. The worst sin was smoking."(Page 56).

Steve also recommended drinking a glass of warm water with honey and lemon before breakfast, which led intuitively to his natural "Gatorade"–like "Electrolyte Workout Formula" for replacing and replenishing essential electrolytes like chloride, potassium and sodium lost through perspiration during training. These water–dissolvable electrolytes determine how much fluid remains inside cells and how much remains outside cells. My buffoonish friends at the gym have christened the workout drink, *"Urineade!"* Another punster calls it "bug juice" because of its honey content. Droll souls!

WORKOUT DRINK
(mixed in a half-gallon container)
•Honey(3 tablespoons)

•Lemon Juice(1/2–cup/dissolves the honey)
•Water(half–gallon)

Measure your mixed ingredients precisely to properly balance the sweet and sour of the honey and lemon. Drink the whole half–gallon of liquid by taking 2–3 sips after each set of weights lifted. This urine–colored drink keeps your energy up throughout your entire workout even though court jesters in the gym will invariably volunteer to refill your half–empty container! John, Pete and Ron *RULE!*

"Something instinctively told me," Steve recounted, "that these nutrients were needed by my body during a workout in order to continue working out at optimum levels. By having the lemon juice and honey, I was able to maintain my body's acid balance, and I had more energy and was able to get much more out of my muscles without tiring them too prematurely. In other words, my muscles would tire out due to genuine muscle fatigue as opposed to some biochemical imbalance."

"I automatically did something correct when I was working out," Steve told official biographer, Chris LeClaire, "I didn't know what I was doing at the time, but I did it instinctively. I used to drink a lot of water, and I'd mix lemon and honey with my water, and that way I was able to replace all the electrolytes that would be lost through perspiration...

"Something instinctively told me 'that's the thing to do, I must do it' and I did. By having lemonade, you know, I alkalized the system and I was able to work out more without my muscles getting too much 'pump' in them too soon. In other words, they would not tire out before they were tired."(Page 69).

§

Speaking of drastic imbalance—mental, physical and spiritual—daytime TV has sunk to the nethermost depths of neuroticism with the introduction to national television of an overweight hack psychologist publicly humiliating overweight people in front of millions of television viewers and giving them to boot profoundly bad advice about how to control or lose their weight and so eliminate their obesity: *"Dr. Phil!"*

Supposedly Phillip C. McGraw(aka *"Dr. Phil"*)is among other unbelievable and unconvincing things America's blunt–talking, get real, get–over–it, in–your–face, tell–it–like–it–is, to–the–point, wake–up–call TV therapist. *Blah, Blah, Blah, Blah!!!!*

By his own website confession, McGraw was a piss–poor psychologist in private practice hanging onto his own practicing psychologist father's coattails! "From the very beginning, it wasn't for me. I didn't have the patience for it," he admits. Now he's a self–described "smart ass" talk–show host who got lucky commercially by weaseling his way into the good graces of Oprah Winfrey! "I think the reason I've enjoyed the response that I have on Oprah's show is because I think that people are ready to hear the truth. I think that they are tired of people blowing smoke..." Well, few blowhards could ever aspire or hope to blow as much smoke—or hot air!—as *"Dr. Phil!"*

"You either get it or you don't," McGraw likes to tell his humiliated television victims. Well, just one look at this puffed up, over–bloated, bombastic charlatan who's roughly only three years my senior should tell almost anyone: *"Dr. Phil"* the **QUACK** sure as **HECK** doesn't get it! So I wonder whether McGraw himself can take the healthy dose of the "truth" which I'm about to dispense:

First off, Quick–Draw–McGraw, you can get real and get over it by getting off that high horse *"DOC-TOR"* Phil bit. Titles of nobility were abolished by the United States Constitution long ago!

That said, I've got only one question for you: where does a bald, jowly and *FAT* pompous *ASS* like yourself *GET OFF* publicly humiliating overweight people in front of millions of television viewers for their obesity? You're a physical *DISGRACE*, so work off your own *FAT* globs before you degrade and denigrate others for theirs!

YOU EITHER GET IT OR YOU DON'T!

§

Diets and willpower meant to control or lose weight don't work, claims McGraw's website. "Overeating" causes obesity! Perpetuating publicly this sort of ***MISGUIDED MISINFORMATION AND STU-PIDITY IS A DEPRAVED AND DISASTROUS DISSERVICE! WHATEVER YOU'RE PROSELY-TIZING SURE AS HECK ISN'T WORKING FOR YOU! YOU'RE A DOPE, "DR. PHIL!"***

Just as *HOW* you exercise is eminently more important than what exercise you do or how much weight you lift, *WHAT* you eat is eminently more important than how *MUCH* you eat!

CORRECT diet combined with willpower–driven exercise ***DOES INDEED WORK—AND PER-MANENTLY—ONCE HABITUATED TO YOUR LIFESTYLE!*** And you ***DO NOT*** have to waste your time and effort ***CONSTANTLY COUNTING CAL-ORIES*** to control or lose weight!

Eat the ***RIGHT FOODS***(meaning without saturated fat, white flour, white sugar)and you *AUTO-*

MATICALLY put yourself on a *REDUCED CAL-ORIE DIET!* You can hardly ever *"over–eat"* the *RIGHT FOODS!* It's so absurdly and ridiculously SIMPLE!

YOU EITHER GET IT OR YOU DON'T!

All you're doing by patronizing this charlatan is helping to finance his opulent lifestyle—like the $7.5–million-dollar Beverly Hills home he recently bought—reportedly "in cash."

How's that for a lead–in to the next chapter about smart supermarket shopping for fitness, health and weight control?

SEVEN:

SUPERMARKET BANKING

"Every time you eat something, think of it as making a deposit in your body's energy bank and remember that too many deposits will result in unwanted fat gain."— Steve Reeves

Bearing in mind these few simple rules of smart nutrition and weight control you can head for your local grocery store or supermarket to shop with complete confidence for the food deposits you'll make to your body's energy bank. And while you're at it—in spite of what that sharper, Nicholas V. Perricone, says—don't forget to make a beeline, as it were, for some healthful honey! To simplify matters shop by major food group from greater to lesser importance nutrition–wise.

§

FOOD! What is it? Well, it's much more than something merely to appease our appetites with. Food is our body's most vital **PROVIDER**. Food provides our bodies not only with energy by way of calories but also all the physiological things our bodies need by way of essential nutrients to build, grow, develop, repair and reproduce themselves. Food sustains our body temperatures and all our bodily processes. Foods differ markedly in the amounts of essential nutrients they provide depending on their source and composition—that is, where they come from and what they're made up of. Getting the right nutrients in the right amounts is why it's so vitally important to pick and choose the right foods to eat!

Keep in view your ideal dietary distribution of 60 percent complex(emphasis)and simple carbohydrates, 20 percent protein and 20 percent fat and confidently set out for the grocery store or supermarket to shop by major food groups for those providers of essential nutrients which our bodies make in amounts not enough for growth and health or not at all .

CARBOHYDRATES

(Fast Fuel)

Carbohydrates(mostly starches and sugars)provide our bodies with their chief source of energy: four calories of energy per gram. Our bodies break down carbohydrates, producing the sugar glucose which is vital to activating the central nervous system, maintaining tissue protein and metabolizing fat.

Starches and sugars comprise the major or complex carbohydrates:

•Starch foods comprise beans, breads, cereals, corn, noodles, pasta, peas, potatoes, whole–grains and yams.

•Sugar foods comprise fruits, honey, maple sugar, milk sugars, sugar cane and vegetables.

Our bodies break down complex carbohydrates into a simpler form to gain that vitally necessary energy fuel: glucose or blood sugar.

Complex carbohydrates also contain indigestible dietary fibers which can be soluble or insoluble:

•Soluble fiber foods comprise apples, barley, beans, brown rice, carrots, citrus fruits, oats, peas, and strawberries. Soluble fiber mixes with food in our stomachs to prevent or reduce the absorption of potentially harmful substances from food by our small intestines. It also binds dietary cholesterol and transports it out of our bodies to prevent it from entering our bloodstreams to accumulate and clog our arteries.

•Insoluble fiber foods comprise bran, vegetables and whole–grains. Insoluble fiber provides roughage which expedites the expulsion of feces, thereby reducing our exposure to potentially harmful substances. Red meat is notorious for literally fermenting inside our intestines!

Ignore the Ignorant. You hear plenty of downright stupid things in gyms—like don't eat rice, potatoes or pasta or you won't develop muscular definition. Even that sharper, Nicholas V. Perricone, absurdly advises against eating cereals, pasta, peas, potatoes and rice(I especially relish *Jasmine* rice). ***BULL!***

Our bodies digest and absorb complex carbohydrates at a rate that maintains healthful levels of glucose already in our blood. Complex carbohydrates get converted to glucose, which is absorbed into our bloodstream through our intestinal wall, activating both our brain cells and red blood cells.

Now, some glucose converted from excess or surplus carbohydrates courses its way to our liver and muscles where it gets stored as glycogen(animal starch)and to fat cells where it gets stored as fat. Any leftover carbohydrates get converted to some amino acids utilized in protein synthesis.

Glycogen and fat comprise the storage or reserve forms of calories for energy:

•Glycogen is our body's auxiliary source of energy—tapped and converted back into glucose whenever our muscles demand more energy for exercise. That's why honey's high–glycogen content in your electrolyte replacement workout drink will keep your energy level up throughout your workout while your contemporaries plop themselves down onto their benches all pooped out between their weight–training sets from fatigue due to exercise fuel depletion(low levels of liver and muscle glycogen—the storage forms of carbohydrates).

•Fat acts as an alternate, backup or substitute source of energy but it's never converted into glucose. That's why you should refrain from consuming excessive complex carbohydrates to minimize any conversion to fat.

Otherwise, foods rich in complex carbohydrates

supply an essential and plentiful source of energy—not to mention vitamins, minerals, some protein and dietary fiber. So don't scrimp on shopping for your complex carbohydrates!

It's the simple sugars contained in refined white sugar form and processed foods which raise levels of glucose in the blood from rapid absorption by the body, triggering the release of the hormone insulin to retard the rising blood sugar levels, resulting in yet another release of chemicals named anti–insulin hormones.

Stick to the simple rules and be careful only about confusing unhealthful white flour products(like cakes, cookies, crackers, doughnuts and white breads) with healthful whole–grains(like brown rice, whole wheat pasta and whole wheat bread)or unhealthful processed and refined white sugar products(like candy, ice cream and soda)with healthful sugar foods(like fresh fruits and honey). And of course eating potatoes does *NOT* translate to eating deep–fried, fast food French fries—high in unhealthy trans fatty acids!

PROTEIN
(Amino Acids)

Proteins provide amino acids for forming body proteins, comprising the structural proteins for building and repairing body tissues and the enzymes for carrying on metabolic processes—in particular those antibodies which help protect against diseases and viruses. Proteins act as chemical messengers, expedite chemical reactions, fight infection, maintain body structure and transport oxygen from the lungs to the body's tissues.

Protein is part and parcel of every body cell. Our body needs a constant supply of protein to repair body cells as they deteriorate. Vital to the blood vessels, muscles, nervous system, organs and skeleton protein is crucial to our bodily growth and development.

Proteins consist of 22 smaller units named amino acids. Thirteen amino acids are made by the human body—synthesized by human cells. Nine essential amino acids must be provided by food protein. Our digestive tract breaks this dietary protein from food into amino acids. Amino acids—once absorbed into the bloodstream and sent to the necessary cells—recombine into the functional proteins our bodies need. Proteins come complete or incomplete:

•Complete(Animal)Proteins contain all 22 amino acids—including all nine essential amino acids our bodies need. Foods providing complete proteins include beef, cheese, chicken, eggs, fish, lamb, milk, pork, shellfish, turkey and yogurt.

•Incomplete(Plant)Proteins contain some but lack all nine essential amino acids but can be combined in your diet to provide all nine essential amino acids. Foods providing incomplete proteins include beans, cereals, grains, lentils, nuts, peas, seeds, soybeans and vegetables. Soy is exceptional because it is the only plant food and complete protein containing all nine essential amino acids—and that's why it makes a superior protein supplement in your daily protein shake! Beans and rice is an excellent combination of plant protein foods providing all nine essential amino acids since either one alone lacks one or more essential amino acids—providing thereby a complete source of protein.

Like carbohydrates, protein provides four calories per gram of energy which the body utilizes as an alternate auxiliary source only if carbohydrate and fat intake is lacking. Getting tapped as an energy source, though, diverts protein from the many critical and unique functions it performs for our bodies—yet another crucial reason why you shouldn't scrimp on consuming your complex carbohydrates!

Ignore the Ignorant! You hear plenty of downright stupid things in gyms—like it's supposed to be advisable or desirable to go out after your workout and eat stacks of fast food burgers for protein replacement! **BULL!**

Since excess amino acids cannot be stored for later use the body destroys them and excretes their by–products. And since our kidneys filter the by–products resulting from the breakdown of protein excessive protein can be harmful to the kidneys. Those by–products can be toxic to the body. Eating excessive protein then adversely and needlessly stresses and taxes the kidneys by overworking them.

With so–called "high–protein" diets your body shifts to a type of metabolism which produces ketones—the presence of which in your blood system causes your blood to become acidic. Persistent acidity can in turn contribute to headaches, irritability, kidney ailments, muscle breakdown, nausea and brittle bones for want of sufficient calcium. Such diets are likely highly deficient in essential nutrients like calcium, potassium and various vitamins.

And since complete protein comes mostly from animal foods excessive protein diets translate to an unhealthy and undesirable intake of cholesterol and saturated fat from certain meats and whole milk dairy products. That's why you'll frequently witness at your gym over time otherwise fit and healthy youth, imitating gullibly their resident bulk–builder's excessively "high–protein" diet, getting not "bigger"—as they witlessly expect—but **FATTER!** A protein intake of only one to two grams per kilogram of body weight is plenty for building muscle mass!

"Protein works and has been around for years," Steve wrote for *All Natural Muscular Development* magazine, "but it does so rather slowly. Amino acids work—after all they should since they are the building blocks of protein—but a person usually has to take so many of them to get any hugely noticeable effect, and the cost of doing so makes this unwise financially...I guess you should ask yourself, will I have a bigger, better and stronger body with whey protein or good old–fashioned milk and egg protein? At the end of the day, protein is still protein and it's not going to do a damn thing for you unless you train hard, eat a well–balanced diet of good wholesome foods, keep your stress levels low, and get plenty of sleep."(December 1997, Volume 34, Number 12, Page 130).

So did Steve ever advocate the so–called "low–carbohydrate" diets so in vogue among today's contemporary bulk–builders? "No," Steve told *Muscle and Fitness* magazine quite bluntly. "I made sure I had plenty of protein and roughage and did plenty of exercise. We didn't have steroids in those days. We had wheat germ, gelatin and brewer's yeast. Some of the advanced people like Vince Gironda took desiccated liver. These were all natural anabolics. A typical breakfast in those days was a pint of orange juice, two tablespoons of Knox gelatin, a tablespoonful of honey, a banana and four raw eggs all blended together. I'd eat at 8 a.m. and train from 9–11. For lunch I'd have cottage cheese, nuts, raisins and a few pieces of fruit in season. For dinner I'd have a huge salad and either a swordfish steak, turkey, tuna or lean ground meat."(May 1983, Page 134). "We mainly lived on fruits and vegetables," Steve reminisced to *Iron Game History* about his youthful "Muscle Beach" days, "and we'd get our protein from cottage cheese and tuna. We ate a lot of cottage cheese. We'd mix cottage cheese with raisins, cottage cheese with carrots, and other things."(December 2000, Volume 6, Number 4, Page 4). "When I was in hard training to put on muscle," he recounted in even further detail, "I would always take my special 'Power Drink'(a meal replacement drink I created)as it was loaded with natural sugars and carbohydrates. I would typically have it for breakfast. I mean, a person could have it at any time, but you could have it for breakfast before your morning workout. I think a person who wanted to lose weight should have their Power Drink for breakfast and lunch, and then for supper have a well–rounded meal consisting of a huge salad(I always prefer rice vinegar and olive oil for my salad dressing, usually a tablespoon of each)and additional protein sources consisting of turkey, fish or chicken, as well as some carbohydrates in the form of whole wheat bread, potatoes, corn, pasta, beans or rice."(***Dynamic Muscle Building***, Page 124).

FAT
(Fatty Acids)

Fats provide the most concentrated source of energy—nine calories per gram of fat as opposed to the four calories per gram of carbohydrate or protein. So our bodies need to ingest only small amounts of fats incorporated sparingly into our diets.

Fats act as a source of stored energy in our bodies. Fats form parts of the membranes surrounding our cells and help blood to clot. Fats cushion our vital organs and insulate our tissues, thereby maintaining our body temperature and protecting us from extreme cold or heat. Digested fats help our bodies transport and absorb from the intestine the fat–soluble vitamins A, D, E and K.

Excess dietary fat is converted to body fat and stored in fat cells. Later, our bodies can tap these fat stores for energy. Unfortunately, the human body's capacity for storing fat is limitless. Because fat takes longer to leave the stomach than either carbohydrates or protein you feel fuller for a longer period of time after eating fat. So we must be extremely careful and cautious about both the amounts and types of fat we ingest. Foods provide essentially three types of fat:

- Monounsaturated
- Polyunsaturated
- Saturated

Depending upon which foods they derive from are fats—just like cholesterol—"good"(beneficial)or "bad"(harmful). So let's clear up all this nonsensical **MALARKEY** about fat and cholesterol—both of which our bodies actually need in correct amounts and types—once and for all!

Animal fats contained in butter, egg yolks, meats, and oils rate high in saturated fats and cholesterol—a chemical substance contained in all animal fat. Vegetable or plant fats contained in avocados, nuts, olives, and certain vegetable oils are rich in unsaturated fat—whether monounsaturated or polyunsaturated. Adding relatively minute amounts of unsaturated fat to your diet is as advisable and desirable as limiting or eliminating from your diet saturated fat. And the crucial reason for making this distinction has to do chiefly with the chemical cholesterol.

Our bodies actually need cholesterol to form cell membranes, protect nerve fibers and produce vitamin D and some hormones which in turn act as chemical messengers coordinating our bodily functions. Since our liver and small intestine make all the cholesterol our bodies need—and since excessive levels of cholesterol in the blood can contribute to certain cancers(of the breast, colon, prostate and uterus), diabetes, heart disease, hypertension and obesity—cholesterol in the diet is nonessential as a nutrient and should be reduced.

Since cholesterol(like fat)is a lipid—an organic compound not soluble in water—it must be transported through the blood by special carriers called lipoproteins, prompting us to distinguish between so-called "good" and "bad" cholesterol:

•High–Density Lipoproteins(HDLs)comprise "good" cholesterol: HDLs remove cholesterol from the walls of arteries and return it to the liver which excretes it as bile—a liquid acid essential to fat digestion.

•Low–Density Lipoproteins(LDLs)comprise "bad" cholesterol: LDLs transport cholesterol from the liver to the cells, clogging the arteries by leaving plaque–forming cholesterol in the artery walls.

Due to this vital distinction: *WE SHOULD CONSUME DIETARY FATS WHICH INCREASE THE LEVELS OF OUR HDLs AND DECREASE THE LEVELS OF OUR LDLs!*

Now we can more astutely distinguish between "good"(unsaturated)and "bad"(saturated)*FAT*:

•Monounsaturated Fats—contained in canola, hazelnut, olive and peanut oils—most beneficially affect blood cholesterol, decreasing the blood level of LDLs("bad" cholesterol)while increasing the blood level of HDLs("good" cholesterol).

•Polyunsaturated Fats—contained in margarine and corn, safflower, soybean and sunflowers oils—can decrease the blood level of HDLs if consumed in excess(greater than ten percent of daily calories).

•Saturated Fats—contained in cocoa butter, coconut oil, doughnuts, ice cream, lard, meat, mozzarella cheese, palm oil, poultry, tropical oil, whole milk—can both decrease the blood level of our HDLs and increase the blood level of our LDLs, posing potential harm to both our heart and blood vessels.

Even *non–dairy creamers* are usually made from coconut oil or palm oil, which are saturated fats mixed with additives.

Two other fats also comprise "good" and "bad" types:

•Omega-3 Fat(good)is an essential polyunsaturated fat which the body cannot make derived chiefly from fish sources—in particular cold–water fish like albacore tuna, herring, lake trout, mackerel, salmon and sardines. Flaxseed provides another excellent source of this essential fat—that's why I add it to my milk–based protein shakes!

•Trans Fats(bad)are formed once vegetable oils get processed into solid margarine or shortening by the process known as partial hydrogenation which can decrease HDL cholesterol levels and increase LDL cholesterol levels in the blood. Baked and fried snack foods made with partially hydrogenated vegetable oil or vegetable shortening(like cakes, chips, cookies, crackers, doughnuts and French fries)most typically contain lots of trans fats.

VITAMINS

Vitamins are organic(carbon)compounds and nutrients needed in small amounts to sustain life; they're essential since they can't be made by the human body and must be ingested from foods or vitamin supplements. Organic components of diets found in everything eaten from animal or plant sources contain small amounts of vitamins which are critical to many vital functions in our bodies. Among their many functions vitamins act as enzymes or enzyme aids(coenzymes)to stimulate bodily reactions since a distinct enzyme starts the process of every reaction. Vitamins enhance the body's use of carbohydrates, proteins and fats. Vitamins are crucial in the formation of blood cells, the genetic material deoxyribonucleic acid(DNA), hormones and nervous system chemicals called neurotransmitters. Excessive vitamin levels in the body can cause serious toxic side effects.

•Fat–soluble vitamins: vitamins A, D, E and K are absorbed with the aid of foods containing fat. So they're dissolvable in fat, stored in fat in the body and transported by fat through the body. They're found in fatty foods. Fat containing these vitamins is broken down by bile—a liquid released by the liver—and the body absorbs the breakdown products and vitamins. Excess amounts of fat–soluble vitamins get stored in the body's fat, kidneys and liver so they don't need to be ingested every day to meet the body's needs.

•Water–soluble vitamins: B1(thiamine), B2(riboflavin), B3(niacin), B6, B12, C(ascorbic acid), biotin, folate(folic acid), pantothenic acid cannot be stored, dissolve in water–based fluids and rapidly exit the body if ingested in greater quantities than the body needs. Foods containing water–soluble vitamins must be eaten daily to replenish the body's needs.

•Antioxidants: vitamins A(in beta-carotene form), C and E are essential to countering the potential harm of chemicals known as free radicals which unchecked make cells more susceptible to cancer–causing substances. Free radicals originating from cigarette smoke and environmental pollutants can convert bodily chemicals to cancer–causing agents.

MINERALS

Minerals are inorganic(carbon–free)compounds and nutrients needed in small amounts to sustain life. Minerals are essential to many parts of the body— particularly the bones—and they make up parts of other crucial compounds like iodine(part of the thyroid hormone)and iron(in blood). Minerals control the balance between acids and bases and maintain the body's fluid balance. Minerals—more stable than vitamins—break down in air and light and dissolve in water. The mineral content of certain foods is affected by the mineral content of the soil in which those foods are grown. Even cooking utensils can add minerals to foods. Minute amounts of metallic elements are essential to the healthy growth of bones and teeth. They also aid cellular activity like blood clotting, enzyme action, muscle contraction and nerve reaction. Ingesting too much minerals can be toxic.

•Major elements: calcium, chlorine, magnesium(important to bones and the normal functioning of muscles and nerves), phosphorus, potassium, sodium and sulfur(part of proteins and vitamins). Calcium and phosphorous are found in skeletal bone, teeth and muscle. Chloride, potassium and sodium are the fluid–regulating electrolytes which also maintain the functioning of the nervous system.

•Trace elements: aluminum, chromium, cobalt, copper, fluoride(essential to bone and teeth development), iodine(part of the thyroid hormones), iron manganese(important part of hemoglobin keeping oxygen in the blood), molybdenum, selenium(part of the important antioxidant, glutathione peroxidase) tin, vanadium and zinc.

•Ultratrace elements: arsenic, boron, nickel and silicon.

To come to the point: get your vitamins and minerals by eating a vast variety of foods—or, in short, a nutritious and well–balanced diet!

§

"And I don't believe in low–fat, no–fat diets," that sharper, Nicholas V. Perricone, told Pat Robertson in his CBN News interview. Well, that depends on the fat you chew! Out of all this *GOBBLEDY–GOOK*, then, I can safely suggest that it's most definitely beneficial to eliminate harmful saturated fat, white flour and white sugar from your daily diet.

Ignore the Ignorant! You hear plenty of downright stupid things in gyms—like it's healthful to eat gobs of fat–striated beef or pork so long as you trim away its visible fat or don't drink fruit juices because of the calories and natural sugars they contain.

JUNK FOODS are *PROCESSED FOODS* providing only *EMPTY CALORIES* since they're loaded with calories derived from saturated fats and refined simple sugars but lack those essential nutrients our bodies need most. Foods containing more calories than nutrients are empty calories.

We've been misled far too long by so–called health and fitness "experts" to believe that the principal culprit to blame for obesity is simply excess calories rather than nutrient–*deficient* calories. Calories in fact are neither more nor less than units of energy—those provided by the food we consume and those utilized by our bodies through our varied activity. Without nutrient–*dense* calories we couldn't even live much less move! And our bodies burn calories to both live and move!

Nutrient–density, incidentally, is simply a measure of nutrients per calorie. And nutrient–dense foods provide more nutrients but less calories while nutrient–deficient foods provide more calories(and/or fat)and less nutrients.

Nutrients found in foods from all the major food groups providing calories remain limited to carbohydrates, protein and fat. Foods also provide vitamins, minerals and water but none of those necessary nutrients provide calories! That's why I recommend supermarket shopping—or energy banking—by major food group distributed among complex carbohydrates(60 percent), protein(20 percent)and fat(20 percent): so you can automatically balance both calories and nutrients in the foods you buy.

Remember that carbohydrates, proteins and fats all provide the body with energy in the form of calories. These nutrients get released from foods during digestion, absorbed into the bloodstream and converted to glucose or blood sugar—which our bodies actually exploit as energy. Unused energy gets stored either as glycogen(the stored form of glucose)in the liver and muscles or as fat. More vitally important than the calories themselves are the nutrients they come from! Cooking food in olive oil(monounsaturated fat) is obviously much more healthful than heaping your salad with creamy dressing or your sandwich with mayonnaise—both saturated, in a sense, with saturated fat!

§

A Word About Watermelon. That sharper, Perricone, lists my two favorite fruits—grapes and watermelon—as foods to "avoid" while listing tomatoes as a food to "enjoy." When in fact both tomatoes and watermelon are major sources of *lycopene*—that so-called *"phyto–chemical"* natural plant substance, powerful antioxidant and carotenoid that's supposed to prevent certain cancers and other ailments like heart disease by neutralizing highly unstable molecules which would otherwise do cell damage; it gives guava, pink and red grapefruit, tomatoes and watermelon their characteristic color as well. Besides being also a source of vitamin C watermelon is one among the fruits least concentrated in both sugar and calories. So it's obviously great for weight–control too!

§

PRACTICAL(NOT PERRICONE)PRESCRIPTION FOR INTELLIGENT NUTRITION AND WEIGHT CONTROL

•Bake, boil, broil, poach, roast, sauté, steam or stir–fry rather than fry food.

• Cook with canola, olive or peanut oil.

•Drain fat from browned meat.

•Drink low–fat(1%-2%), nonfat or skim milk.

•Drink one to two glasses of red wine daily—preferably Cabernet Sauvignon because of its polyphenols(chemicals which reduce the production of a certain protein to blame for the build–up of harmful fat deposits within the walls of our arteries).

•Drink fruit, tomato and vegetable juices. These days my favorite beverage of choice is 100% grapefruit juice.

•Dump your butter, margarine and mayonnaise(I lightly spread blueberry preserves on whole wheat toast and fatless honey mustard on whole wheat sandwich bread). For that matter, honey mustard beans and honey mustard salad dressings are terrific too!

•Eat lots of beans. Black beans are best. Even canned pork and beans are low–fat.

•Eat cereals with at least 4 grams of fiber and less than 5 grams of sugar per serving. Of the name brands I prefer Product 19, Special K, Total and Wheaties.

•Eat fat–free or low–fat cheese(5 grams of fat per ounce or less).

•Eat low–fat crackers.

•Eat canned fruit packed in its "own juice" or with "no sugar added."

•Eat fresh fruit, light ice cream with 5 grams of fat per scoop or one-half cup or less, 100 percent juice bars, sherbet or frozen low–fat or nonfat yogurt for desserts.

•Eat leaner cuts of meat(loin and round cuts). Sirloin and tenderloin taste best; round is too tough. Canadian is preferable to regular bacon.

•Eat luncheon meats with 2 grams of fat per serving or less. Avoid all hot dogs.

•Eat pasta without fat–filled stuffing like ravioli or tortellini.

•Eat more fish(avoid breaded or pre–fried), chicken and turkey(avoid processed cuts like turkey bologna) instead of beef and pork. Eat mostly fish and seafood if you want to cut body–fat fast.

•Eat broth–based soups like chicken noodle, minestrone and vegetable. Avoid cream soups.

•Eat canned tuna packed in spring water.

•Eat whole–grain breads with 2 grams of fat per slice maximum, including whole wheat bagels, English muffins and pita bread.

•Economize by bulk–buying frozen instead of exorbitantly high–priced fresh produce. Frozen fruits and vegetables(like blueberries, carrots, corn, lima beans, peas, peaches, raspberries, spinach and strawberries) retain their nutrients preserved by the fast–freeze process—often longer than fresh produce exposed to air and light(breaking down their vitamin content) long past their harvest date, though in–season fresh fruits and vegetables contain the highest levels of nutrients.

•Eliminate from your diet all meat and its attendant calorie–saturated animal fat(including even leaner meats like chicken and turkey breast)altogether if you want to cut body–fat super–fast! That simply means turning at least semi–vegetarian though you can still get your requisite protein from non–animal sources like brewer's yeast, gelatin, soy along with egg whites to complete your intake of essential amino acids.

•Flavor food with citrus juices, herbs, spices and wine without fat.

•Mix bean, pasta, rice and vegetable dishes(like casseroles, chili, soup, spaghetti sauce and stir–fries) with small amounts of lean meat.

•Skim fat from soups and stews.

•Snack on nuts or seeds.

•Steer clear of supermarket aisles displaying biscuits, cake, candy, chips, cookies, crackers, croissants, doughnuts, ice cream, pastries, scones and soda. ***DON'T EVEN THINK ABOUT IT!***

•Trim skin from poultry.

•Trim visible fat from meat.

Steve's weight–loss prescription is exceptionally simple and practical: "I think a person who wanted to lose weight should have their Power Drink for breakfast and lunch, and then for supper have a well–rounded meal consisting of a huge salad(I always prefer rice vinegar and olive oil for my salad dressing, usually a tablespoon of each)and additional protein sources consisting of turkey, fish or chicken, as well as some carbohydrates in the form of whole wheat bread, potatoes, corn, pasta, beans or rice."(***Dynamic Muscle Building***, Page 124).

As for "dieting hints," Steve offered these general guidelines from his book, ***Power Walking***(1982):

•Decrease caloric intake.

•Eat your largest meal at lunch time.

•Learn to eat slowly and chew thoroughly.

•Limit portions of food at meals to one average serving.

•Never take second helpings.

•Omit or drastically restrict free fats—butter, margarine, mayonnaise, salad oils, cooking fats. Sufficient fat is present in lean meats, fish, poultry, eggs, and cheese to ensure adequate use of the fat–soluble vitamins A, D, E, and K.

•Omit or drastically restrict free sweets—jelly, jam, honey, syrups, sugar, candy, pies, pastries, and most other desserts.

•Restrict or eliminate intake of alcoholic beverages.

•Eat a good breakfast and never skip a meal.

•Never use food as a reward.

•Learn to practice moderation.

EIGHT:

INSIGHT INTO THE STEVE REEVES DIET

"Do you not know that your body is a temple of the holy Spirit within you, whom you have from God, and that you are not your own? For you have been purchased at a price. Therefore, glorify God in your body."—1 Corinthians 6: 19–20

STAY FIT(AND HOT)FOR LIFE

Thanks to the contribution of firsthand information made available by Steve's widow, Deborah Engelhorn–Reeves–Stewart, I'm profoundly pleased to provide these modest insights into the daily diet and supplements of **STEVE REEVES**:

COLD–WEATHER DISHES

- Chicken with rice
- Chili with beans and cornbread
- Cod Filets(breaded)
- Corned Beef with cabbage
- Lasagne
- Pot Roast
- Roast Beef with potatoes
- Roast Chicken with potatoes
- Roast Pork with potatoes
- Roast Turkey with potatoes
- Spaghetti
- Swordfish Steaks(breaded)

HOT–WEATHER DISHES

- Chicken chunks in green salad
- Cottage cheese(1% fat)with cranberry sauce(whole berry)
- Cottage cheese with jello
- Cottage cheese with tuna
- Proscuitto with avocado, cantaloupe(slices), mozzarella cheese and tomato(one of Steve's favorites!)
- Soup with green salad
- Tuna in green salad

SIDE DISHES
(Steamed)

- Artichokes
- Asparagus
- Broccoli
- Cauliflower

- Potatoes
- Rice
- Salads
- Steve's own salad dressing: ½ Extra Virgin Cold–Pressed Olive Oil and ½ Nakano Seasoned Rice Vinegar

BEVERAGES

- Malibu Sunrise: cranberry juice(1/3), orange juice(1/3 fresh squeezed), water(1/3)
- Milk(1% fat often with dinner)

DESSERTS

- Apple Pie a la mode
- Ice Cream
- Pumpkin Pie
- Strawberry Pie(homemade: strawberry jello and fresh strawberries in graham pie crust)with Cool Whip

FAVORITE RESTAURANT MEAL

- Prime Rib
- Salad with Ranch dressing

MEXICAN DISHES

- Bean and Beef(shredded)Burrito
- Tostado(occasional)

SUPPLEMENT

High Potency Multivitamin/Mineral:
- Vitamins A, B(complex), C, E(gel)
- Calcium
- Garlic(capsule)
- Ginseng
- Glucosamine Sulfate
- Iron
- Kelp
- Phosphorous
- Potassium Glucosinate
- Selenium

•Aspirin(81 mg, preventative)

COLD REMEDY

•Whole Wheat Toast(2 slices spread liberally with extra virgin olive oil and garlic slices)

•Vitamin C/Zinc(lozenge)

BREAKFAST PROTEIN DRINK FORMULA

(Precursor To The "Steve Reeves Power Drink")

•Orange Juice(12 ounces, freshly squeezed)

•Banana(1 whole)

•Eggs(2 raw)

•Bee Pollen(1 teaspoon, fresh)

•Honey(1 teaspoon)

•*Knox* Gelatin(2 packets)

•Oats(1/8 cup, old–fashioned rolled)/Exchangeable with Wheat Germ

•Skim Milk(1/8 cup, powdered)

•Soy Protein(1/8 cup, powdered)

•Wheat Germ(1/8 cup)

When he was but 23 Steve specified his juicer power–drink ingredients this way: "I pour into this electric juicer one pint of orange juice, four raw eggs, two bananas and two tablespoons of honey. When these are thoroughly mixed it represents my breakfast."(***Dynamic Muscle Building***, Page 140).

In his almanac–length book, *Steve Reeves: His Legacy In Films(2003)*, Dave Dowling recounted how Steve maintained his healthful and wholesome regimen even while busily engaged working on major motion picture film sets:

•"Long before it was fashionable, he(Steve)ate sprouts, flowers and sunflower seeds. One day he ate an orchid in front of me!" Actress Debbie Reynolds reminisced about Steve's participation in their movie, *Athena*(1954/Pages 2-8).

•"To maintain his physique during the filming(of

Hercules, 1957), Steve…also made sure his diet consisted of beef or chicken, pasta, a quart of tomato juice or milk, and some fruit."(Pages 3-11).

•"With food," Steve recollected about his movie, *The White Warrior*(1959), "I would have a large steak with two eggs on top three times a day as well as a liter of goat's milk each day."(Pages 5-11).

•"After that," Steve recollected about his movie, *Thief of Baghdad*(1961), "I decided to eat only cheese, tuna, and bread for the rest of the filming. I'm also convinced that yogurt made from camel's milk has an energy–giving ingredient that can't be found anywhere else in the normal human diet. I'm not kidding when I say I'd walk a mile for a camel, just as long as it gave milk."(Pages 10-13).

•"I remember that he(Steve)drank a lot of fruit and vegetable juices," recalled Italian actor and frequent Reeves co–star, Mimmo Palmara. "He used vitamin and protein supplements, but what I noticed most, was that he drank lots of tomato juice. He was against the use of anabolic steroids and never considered taking them."(Pages 16-17).

From **Dynamic Muscle Building** other amongst Steve's daily nutritional practices comprised:

•"For lunch I drink one quart of goat's milk, which I get fresh every day, and also eat a handful of figs."(Page 140).

•"Well, later in the day, about an hour before my dinner, I drink a pint or a quart of fresh carrot juice that I make from fresh carrots and mix with my juicer."(Page 140).

•"For dinner I usually have one pound of steak, or plenty of fish, or fowl, with two large baked potatoes, or plenty of mashed potatoes, together with a big salad of vegetables, tomatoes and cottage cheese."(Page

140).

•"I was careful to eat a well balanced diet consisting of a large amount of high–protein food, large green salads, baked potatoes, a lot of beef—mainly steak. My diet included raw eggs, honey, bananas, cheese, dried and fresh fruits, and all wholesome foods which gave me energy and muscular bodyweight."(Page 143).

NINE:

THE TRAVESTY OF STEROIDAL BULK–BUILDING (IN STEVE'S OWN WORDS TO THE MASS MEDIA)

"It(Building The Classic Physique—The Natural Way)was written for the natural bodybuilder, so druggies need not apply, if you get my drift."—Steve Reeves

"The only steroid I ever took was brewer's yeast," Steve once told Armand Tanny, profiling him for *Muscle & Fitness* magazine(May 1983, Page 118). That pretty much says it all once you studiously consider the incomparable and phenomenal physique he built without resort to any kind of drugs, much less steroids. "I believe," Steve jested, "that if a man doesn't have enough male hormones within himself to build his body he should take up something like ping–pong."(***Dynamic Muscle Building***, Page 15). When it came to the controversial subject of steroids in bodybuilding, though, Steve never minced his words:

Flex
(February 1993)

•"I think the introduction of steroids was the worst thing to ever happen to the field of bodybuilding. To me, the bodybuilders of today look like clones. In other words, they all look like they're out of the same mold. Sure, some of them have blonde hair, some have black hair, some have fair skin and others dark skin, some are shorter and some are taller, but all of them look like they were stamped out of the same mold. And that's the sort of bloated–tissue look caused by steroids. In my day,…People were individuals at that time. Now they work out with the same routine, with the same steroids and, as a result, they've come to look too much like each other. Furthermore, they waste their lives training all the time. There's more to life than training, you know what I mean? And when they're off the drugs, they look like nothing…In my day, bodybuilding was a health–oriented activity instead of a drug–oriented sport. Steroids surfaced in bodybuilding, I think, because people wanted to take the 'easy' way to get to the top. When one guy took the easy way and got some results, somebody else did it and it just snowballed from there. Even the judges encouraged it by giving out trophies to the people with the 'biggest' legs, not the 'best–developed' legs; the 'biggest' arms, not the 'best–developed,' and so on. It just got out of hand. If everybody got off steroids, I think the quality of physiques would improve, because all of the athletes would be competing at their ideal weight."(Pages 112-113).

All Natural Muscular Development
(May 1997, Volume 34, Number 5)

•"I've always loved bodybuilding. But the drugs turned me off. I've been against steroids from the start. I saw what they had produced: Guys with biceps larger than their heads, blocky bodies, big bellies and wide waists. So many of those guys still don't have calves. Bodybuilders should do their shopping at the health food store. Not with a doctor's prescription at drugstores. The best of those guys won't live to be 60, let alone 70!"(Page 205).

•"I have a hard time hanging around the steroid bodybuilders. So aggressive; they give off really bad vibes."(Page 206).

•"They're(drugs)giving bodybuilding such a bad name. That's so unfair to bodybuilders who train the natural way. We've all got to pitch in and try to reverse the trend!"(Page 206).

•"The introduction of steroids was the worst thing to happen to bodybuilding...They all have the bloated–tissue look and the coarse, pimply skin associated with steroids."(Page 206).

•"When the drugged bodybuilders go off their steroids they don't look that great either...In my day bodybuilding was a health–oriented activity. Today it's strictly a drug thing."(Page 206).

•"As a bodybuilder you should be shopping at the local health–food store—not with prescriptions at the drugstore."(Page 206).

All Natural Muscular Development
(August 1997, Volume 34, Number 8)

•"It is my belief, if we're ever going to get steroids out of the sport of bodybuilding, that we get rid of the 'size for size's sake mentality' of the judges at these contests. And by that I mean, we must alter their judging criteria. I've worked out a proportion chart that takes into account such factors as height, weight and bone density and circumference, so that your measurements should be proportionate and symmetrical, not just big and bloated. If this was the standard for the prejudging portion of the contest, then suddenly it would no longer behoove a bodybuilder to take a steroid or growth hormone—which has a systemic(as opposed to local)effect that could thereby ruin his symmetry."(Page 104).

•"You've got to step back and take a look at what's going on here; I'm saying 'Pro health, anti–drugs,' and you're either for me or against me on this. If these other people are saying things against what I'm saying, then just what is it they're actually saying? And whose side are you on—The side that says 'don't take drugs, make your body a thing of beauty of form and function, so that you can look great well into the prime of your life?' Or those that say 'take drugs, lie to the public about it—and maybe you'll live to see 50 years of age.' The choice is yours."(Page 208).

All Natural Muscular Development
(November 1997, Volume 34, Number 11)

•"If you want to look like something out of a freak show, then I'm afraid your mind set has less to do with it than chemistry."(Page 148).

All Natural Muscular Development
(February 1998, Volume 35, Number 2)

• "The classic physique—as contrasted with the steroid–bloated physique—reflects a concern with attention to detail."(Page 178).

Ironman
(February 1999, Volume 58, Number 2)

• "Bodybuilding has been completely corrupted by steroids, and steroids are the worst thing to come along since I don't know what. And the guys look like clones! There aren't any individuals left. Bodybuilding should be health–oriented, not drug–oriented. People are dropping dead left and right, and that's insane. I never put any drug in my body to enhance anything, and I think I did pretty damned well."(Page 178).

In a tribute for *Teleport-City.com*, Keith Allison wrote, "Reeves never got that grotesque, 'veins a–poppin' artificial Big Poppa Pump look that comes from relying heavily on 'the juice' as it's known to some people. Steroids. As a product of natural development and healthy living, Steve's build, while most definitely massive, was never freakish or absurd the way a lot of bodybuilders look these days."

"Steve Reeves," Fred Fornicola wrote for *NaturalStrength.com*, "with his classically sculpted body winning such notable titles as Mr. World, Mr. America and Mr. Universe has contributed so much to the iron game that it is a shame that today's bodybuilders don't follow the path that he worked so hard at paving over 50 years ago. If you were to take away all the steroids, growth hormones and whatever else illegally that produce the freakish bodies that are around today they wouldn't be able to hold a candle to Mr. Steve Reeves...I hope that more people would take pride and have the dedication that Steve had. Today's bodybuilders are not concerned with training hard and progressively; they are more concerned with getting their hands on good drugs to produce their physique. I suggest taking on the Herculean task of working hard, brief and intensely to produce a natural and long lasting physique."

Or as *Outsports.com* put it, "Reeves had a classic physique in the days before steroids were everywhere."

"Since we have these promises, beloved, let us cleanse ourselves from every defilement of flesh and spirit, making holiness perfect in the fear of God."—2 Corinthians 7:1

TEN:

CONTEMPORARY BULK–BUILDING— ADVANCED AND MODERN OR DEADLY AND SUICIDAL?

"Competitive bodybuilding is the least healthy of all sports. On contest days, some bodybuilders are very close to death."— **Anonymous Former Bodybuilder**

Once at the **Berkeley YMCA** gym where I used to train and work out, I overheard its resident bulk–builder denigrating what he disparagingly referred to as the *"old school"* bodybuilders and their supposedly obsolete, outmoded and outdated nutritional and training practices, insinuating so imperiously that he and the likes of his contemporary bulk–builder ilk monopolized superior, all–omniscient knowledge and wisdom by virtue of its being immediate and modern. Contemporary bulk–building, he stupidly implied, surpassed classic bodybuilding simply because anything of the present which was current and topical supposedly surpassed anything of the past which was automatically old–fashioned and out of style. If then you mistakenly think that anything of the distant past is necessarily passé then **THINK AGAIN!** When it comes to promoting true and total fitness, health and longevity, I'm here to tell you that classic bodybuilding surpasses contemporary bulk–building in every respect! Why? Once you honestly contrast the two opposing schools you readily discover that while the old school is still alive and thriving the supposedly superior new school is **DEAD AND DYING OFF IN DROVES!!!!** So if you're still all atwitter to witlessly make a stupid practice of patently detrimental *"new school"* habits then do so at your own risk and peril!

"I must also give credit to Jack LaLanne," Steve confided to *Muscle and Fitness* magazine, "who developed many new bodybuilding techniques and equipment I found so helpful. I think he was the first person to use the incline bench."(May 1983, Page 127).

"I got the idea for formulating these 'classic' proportions from looking at Jack LaLanne," Steve recounted in his bodybuilding book, "who had a big chest and a small waist—in fact, Jack has a 20–inch difference between the measurement of his chest and waist."

Given Steve's reverent admiration for him it's most telling to note that *JACK LALANNE*—the reputed *"Godfather of Fitness"* who ranked tenth in the Mr. USA contest of 1948—in September 2004 turned 90 years old! Steve ranked second in the very same contest after Clarence Ross. In January 2000, I turned 50!

Dead men are supposed to tell no tales. Dead natural classic physique bodybuilders of the so–called *"old school"* on the other hand tell a most definite—and definitive—tale of true health, vitality and *LONGEVITY*. Let their statistical, relative, high–mortality life–spans speak convincing volumes in and of themselves:

- Eugen Sandow(1867–1925): 58
- Bobby Pandur(1876–1920): 44
- Adolph Pitz(1879–195?): 71-?
- John Garon(1886–195?): 64-?
- Charles Atlas(1893–1972): 79
- Ernest Cadine(1893–1978): 85
- Bob Hoffman(1898–1985): 87
- Sigmund Klein(1902–1987): 85
- Charles Rigoulot(1903–1962): 59
- Tony Sansone(1905–1987): 82
- Bert Goodrich(1906–1991): 85(Mr. America, 1939)
- John Grimek(1910–1998): 88(Mr. America, 1940/1941)
- John Terpak(1912–1993): 81
- Sam Loprinzi(1913–1996): 83
- Walt Baptiste(1915–2001): 86
- Steve Stanko(1916–1978): 62(Mr. America, 1944)
- Roland Essmaker(1916–2002): 86

- Juan Ferraro(1918–1958): 40
- Vince Gironda(1918–1997): 79
- Melvin Wells(1919–1994): 75
- Bob McCune(1921–2002): 81
- Kimon Voyages(1922–1989): 67
- Paul Novak(1923–1999): 76
- John Farbotnik(1925–1998): 73(Mr. America, 1950)
- Floyd Page(1926–1963): 37
- Jack Delinger(1926–1994): 68(Mr. America, 1949)
- **STEVE REEVES**(1926–2000): 74(Mr. America, 1947)
- Billy Hill(1928–1979): 51
- Eric Pedersen(1928–1990): 62
- Artie Zeller(1930–1999): 69
- Jim Dardanis(1930?–1991): 61?
- Eddie Silvestre(1931–2000): 69
- Leonard Chambers(1932–1955): 23
- Chuck Sipes(1932–1993): 61
- Dave Sheppard(1932–2000): 68
- Mike Sill(1934–1994): 60
- Tom Sansone(1935–1974): 39
- John Tristram(1935–1985): 50
- Don Peters(1936–2001): 65
- Vern Weaver(1937–1993): 56
- Sig Latschkowski(1939–2000): 61
- Jesse "Rock" Stonewall(1940–1994): 54
- Don Ross(1946–1995): 49
- Dave Johns(1948–1986): 38
- Gene Massey(1949–1975): 26
- Mike Mentzer(1951–2001): 50
- Ray Mentzer(1953–2001): 48
- Ron Teufel(1957–2002): 45
- Denny Gable(195?–2000): 50?

• Chris Stimson(1970–2000): 30

This is by no means an exhaustive list. Nor does it account for complete circumstances of deaths or low–mortality anomalies. There is nonetheless one unquestionable conclusion: all told, the **OLDER** the *"school"* of bodybuilder the **LONGER–LIVED** since total fitness, health and longevity were persistently emphasized and never separated from natural, drug–free bodybuilding.

"The Golden Age of bodybuilding spanned from the 1940s through the 1970s," wrote Ken O'Neill in an article for *Dolfzine Online Fitness* titled, ***Bodybuilding's Mythic Hero: Reclaiming the Image***. "Two focuses of training permeated the time: 1)health, strength and fitness; and 2)refined, mature development of aesthetic muscular development. Compared to today's Steroid Age and its standards of excellence, The Golden Age of bodybuilding can easily be considered a grassroots age of innocence...

"The Golden Age was steroid–free, and bodybuilding was natural. The longevity of competitive years was greater, and for good reason: the physiques of the heroes of the Golden Age were the result of years of sustained training. But, as steroids entered the picture, became more readily available and more powerful, training achievement could be obtained in a few years. Steroids speed up the development process, but they also shorten the duration of a bodybuilder's career.

"Bodybuilding, up until the use of steroids, was a culture of athletes who trained the natural way, and a culture whose heroes were people who believed in developing their potential without the use of drugs. They were heroes whose achievements and way of living were admired because they offered a beam of healthy, guiding light and encouragement for others."

ELEVEN:

STEVE'S IMPASSIONED PLEAS FOR SANITY IN BODYBUILDING (In His Own Words)

"I've read too many articles that were pure B.S. when it came to giving real muscle building advice, with some 'champion' indicating that some type of exercise, or some new magical supplement was responsible for putting on, in some cases, over 40 pounds of muscle—when it was obvious to anybody with eyes that this fellow made the gains through altering his body chemistry with steroids, growth hormone and/or other such 'bodybuilding' drugs."—Steve Reeves

STAY FIT(AND HOT)FOR LIFE

All Natural Muscular Development
(June 1997, Volume 34, Number 6, Page 208)

"I've always loved bodybuilding—real bodybuilding, that is. And it has bothered me that the word 'bodybuilding' is now synonymous with illegal drug use—rather than health and fitness...I just got tired of seeing all of the steroid–bloated guys on stage calling themselves 'bodybuilders.' I mean it's really bad for the game. In my day, the most risky thing you would take would be Knox Gelatin powder! So much of bodybuilding has become drug–oriented, that the mind set has become 'Well, if so and so is using this type of drug, then I've got to inject myself with that drug, too!'...The whole situation seems ludicrous to me, particularly since the name of the game is building a big, muscular, proportionate, balanced, symmetrical physique that is pleasing to the eye and geared for functional ability—and you can accomplish all of this without drugs. In fact, in my view, the quality of muscle is better if you don't take the drugs, as the drugs seem to cause you to retain water which obscures your definition(which is why there is such rampant diuretic abuse among the 'champions'). If you build your physique naturally, you'll find that you don't bloat up and look soft—the way many of these guys do until they finally tense their muscles(and then they start rippling!). When these guys are relaxed, most of them look like they don't work out; their stomachs protrude, their shoulders droop and they just look unhealthy. I just got tired of seeing this pass for bodybuilding, particularly since I've seen what real bodybuilding is capable of, and I became embarrassed at what has happened to this great and noble activity. I know, for example, that the sport is capable of much more than that; that a real bodybuilder can truly be a role model to today's youth, and not simply a walk-ing drug store or a guy who knows where you can buy illegal drugs the cheapest. My wish is that real bodybuilding can come back again. I think, 20 years from now, people will look back upon these 'dark ages' of bodybuilding and, if they're feeling charitable, per-haps they will consider this period as having been an 'experiment' of sorts to see what the human body was capable of withstanding chemically—and to what dimensions it could swell up. But they certainly will not look back on this era of the druggie as being in any way a healthy thing, and it certainly isn't a long–term thing. It's simply an experiment like they've con-ducted with animals. Being a rancher, as well as a bodybuilder, I'm used to being around animals and, I must say, these drug–filled bodybuilders remind me of the steers that I've seen going to market. All the steers that go into the feed lots have a little pel-let of steroid put in their ear, so that they'll fatten up better and gain more weight and sell for more money(which is another reason why it's not a good idea to have too much beef these days!). And, in some respect, this is what has happened in bodybuilding; the guys have put aside their humanity in order to become prize steers. They're no longer concerned with building a human body to its ultimate potential—be-cause in some instances they actually take in animal hormones in addition to their usual steroids. They're more interested in developing 'freaky mass'—with the emphasis legitimately on the 'freak' element(as in 'freak show')...It really is insane. I mean, how many bodybuilders have—literally—dropped dead or ended up in the hospital from using these drugs?...Ask your-self—all of the attendant health risks aside—what is this telling our youth? I'll save you the thought:

it's telling them that it's okay to be all form and no substance. And, worse still, it's telling them to cheat. As an American, this distresses me considerably, as I've always considered us one of the more moral countries on the face of the earth, and not one that openly condones such unethical actions...I'm interested in seeing bodybuilding return to truly being a form of natural art; of taking a human body to its highest natural limit while still adhering to aesthetic guidelines, in a very health–oriented manner. The alternative to this is the freak show, like you might see at a circus midway. Today's druggie bodybuilder can now stand on stage as the 'puffy, swollen man,' right next to the bearded lady, and the dog–faced boy. I could go on and on as to why the druggie bodybuilders are anathema to real bodybuilding, from often looking fat and out of shape in clothes; to being winded after carrying their suitcase a block and a half...to a host of medical disorders and contraindications that seem to plague many of the 'champions'...I'm for natural bodybuilding—period. Its results last longer and, in the final analysis, health and longevity are what it's all about. I'm presently 70 years of age and still put in a full day's work, six days a week on my ranch. I also take the time to train in Classic Physique style three days per week. I'm not sure that many of the so–called 'champions' of today would be able to put in a full day's work on my ranch and do my thrice weekly workouts. And, I dare say, fewer still will live to see 60 years of age."

All Natural Muscular Development
(July 1997, Volume 34, Number 7, Page 104)
"...the comments you hear at your gym are typical from guys who are selling you something—particularly drugs. They don't care for my message, be-

cause there's no stake in it for them. They make their money from convincing young, impressionable body-builders that they need steroids and other such drugs to be successful. This is a disgrace and these guys shouldn't be just run out of your gym, but out of the country. There's absolutely no place for people who try to make their living by exploiting our youth and sell-ing them harmful substances. I want people to get back to basics—health and fitness for a healthier, longer life. I would take issue with the charge of my 'taking bodybuilding back 40 years,' in fact, I'm tak-ing steps to advance it and move it forward because the people involved in it today have killed the sport. My vision for it is one of health—not of competitors dying after contests...Anyone who says 'we're going backwards with this natural bodybuilding thing,' is endorsing drug use and is only one rung above the drug pusher in my book. Besides, since when is hav-ing a concern with health a backwards step? These people—the ones responsible for the direction body-building has fallen into—have set it back. Health is the most important part of bodybuilding. Looking good is great, but you must have your health with it. You can't have a beautiful Cadillac or Jaguar with an engine that is incapable of taking you out of your driveway...I don't have a lot of respect for the druggie bodybuilders; bodybuilding used to represent hard work, dedication, persistence, perseverance, intel-ligence—in terms of knowing what to eat and what not to eat; how to train and how not to train; think-ing about recovery within the normal limitations of the human body. But now all bets are off; you simply stick a needle in and do some half–assed workout. Or worse still, with Growth Hormone, I'm told that you don't even have to work out—you simply take your shot and can even sit on the sofa and put on lean tissue—indiscriminately, mind you, but you're growing muscle nevertheless..."

AN OPEN LETTER
TO ARNOLD SCHWARZENEGGER
FROM STEVE REEVES

(*All Natural Muscular Development* Website)

"Dear Arnold:

"As you are well aware, the state of bodybuilding is in crisis. Competitors are killing themselves taking drugs that they believe they need to win shows that ultimately count for nothing in either their careers or their lives.

"I know that you love the sport of bodybuilding as much as I do, because you grew up in an era when being a bodybuilding champion meant something. It stirred heroic and noble images in your young mind of how a man could and should look and how vibrant and virile such a man could be. I know because these were the same images that first caused me to pick up a barbell and to seek to better not only my physique, but my life through physical culture(healthful living and bodybuilding).

"Bodybuilding—real bodybuilding—is what I've just described. It can, and has, proven to work wonders in creating real men of substance, as opposed to what it's now become—a creator of men of real substance–abuse. It can and has opened doors—particularly to you and me. We both went on to enjoy successful careers in film and made substantial sums of money, directly as a result of the physical benefits that our bodybuilding training provided.

"And that is why I am now appealing to you to join forces with me and provide a voice that will be heard by the governing authorities in bodybuilding. The steroids and drug use has to stop and it will not stop as long as we condone its use by turning a blind eye to it. I was out of the game for 40 years; I turned my back on competitive bodybuilding because I couldn't bear to watch it become overrun by drug pushers, publishers and promoters who don't give a damn about the welfare of either the sport or the athletes who participate in it, and whose sole concern lies in selling fraudulent nutritional supplements, inferior equipment, and dispensing bogus training advice and selling tickets to bodybuilding events.

"I wish to appeal to the young, star–struck youth within you that first became enraptured by the real bodybuilding experience. You've mentioned that both myself and, more importantly for you, Reg Park, were your heroes while you were growing up in Austria. Reg Park was a great champion, just as you were. But where are the great role models for today's youth? What do you see in today's 'champions' that personifies the attributes of a champion? Where is the grace under pressure? Where is the giving back to the community? Where is the one current bodybuilding champion that you would want to instruct your children?

"And this isn't the fault of the athletes, they're simply trying to achieve and maintain a highly artificial standard of muscle development that is not natural and definitely not enduring. And, if the muscle you build only stays with you as long as you're getting your synthetic hormone shots, what good is it?

"As the promoter, along with your long–time friend, Jim Lorimer, of what is generally considered the best bodybuilding contest in existence, the Arnold Schwarzenegger Classic, you have the power to lead by example. Despite what you read in the Weider magazines, your show is the king of the hill—not the

Olympia. You know it, Jim Lorimer knows it, the bulk of the competitors know it and, more importantly, the IFBB knows it.

"The reason I know that you are still as enthusiastic about bodybuilding as I am is simple: you could have turned your back on your roots the minute you became one of Hollywood's highest paid actors, but you didn't do that. After all, you've earned the right after years and years of gut–busting workouts to walk into the sunset with your seven Mr. Olympia trophies and retire from the sport altogether, content in the knowledge that your inspiration would serve to fuel the workouts of several generations of new bodybuilders the world over. Instead, you continued to support, promote and herald the benefits of bodybuilding for all people. The cynics will say that you did it to make a buck, but the wise know better; one film would yield you the equivalent of 40 years worth of these contests, and yet you still continue to promote them. That can only be explained by one thing—a genuine interest in the sport. I salute you for that, so don't let these fanatics trample underfoot the sport that you've been an integral part of and helped to sustain all these years. They've ridden on your coattails long enough, now it's up to you to take control of the future of this sport.

"What am I suggesting? Simply this: Insist that the IFBB mandate drug testing(and real drug testing for real bodybuilding drugs, not the joke of 'cocaine' and 'nubane' they tried to pass off as bodybuilding 'drug testing' at last year's Mr. Olympia)in all of their shows. At the very least, you can insist that your show is drug tested. The IFBB will listen to you; not only do you put substantial money in their pockets by sanctioning fees, but without question you have been their most eloquent spokesman. Failing this, form your own federation; one that has new, objective, quantifiable standards for building—not the biggest physique or the 'freakiest'—but the best proportioned, most inspirational and the healthiest.

"Arnold, let's work together to put this derailed train back on the tracks and take this sport back to the glory and prestige it once enjoyed and can enjoy again. It won't help us personally, we're no longer competing, but it can be beneficial to the thousands of bodybuilders yet to compete; those who are just now coming along and who will be competing in the years to come.

"Let's give them a sport that has integrity and honor—and a method of training that will not only give them wonderful physiques, but also provide them with a lifetime of health and vitality."

"Yours Sincerely,"

Steve Reeves

STEVE "HERCULES" REEVES
BODYBUILDING LEGEND
JOINS MUSCULAR DEVELOPMENT

(*All Natural Muscular Development* Website)

"For over 30 years I've remained silent and just watched the transition that bodybuilding has made. And in my opinion, and in the opinions of many who have talked to me, bodybuilding, as it's practiced and promoted today, is dying—and dying fast.

"Well, it's a good thing! Never in my life would I have imagined that such a terrific sport would be filled with so–called 'champions' who are held up as heroes and adulated for physiques that are built with drugs. What kind of 'real' bodybuilding champion is that?

"Since when did a distinction need to be made

between a 'natural' bodybuilder and 'chemical body-builder'? When I built my body, you were a bodybuild-er—period! And you did it without drugs, by train-ing hard, eating right and getting the right amount of rest.

"It disturbs me to no end that today's muscle mag-azines are filled with stories on this–and–that cham-pion's routine, when all the while the average man and woman are misled because these same maga-zines won't dare print the truth! And the truth is that these 'champions' built their physiques after spending tens of thousands of dollars on steroids, growth hor-mone, insulin and whatever else happens to be the latest rage.

"The public has been deceived for too long and it's time someone takes a stand. I will!

"I want you to go to any newsstand during any given month and you'll find these same muscle maga-zines with cover blurbs and articles about the latest drugs. Open them up and you'll find page after page about drugs, how to take them and what to avoid. All this is the lie of supposedly giving their readers the information they say they want to know!

"Recently, someone showed me a magazine put out by a young man in Colorado, and I was shocked. Un-believably, bodybuilding is the only 'sport' that has a magazine devoted to drugs! And this magazine pro-motes this character they call 'the guru,' who answers your most-asked drug–related questions.

"After seeing photos of this fella, it makes you wonder; if drugs were so good, why didn't they work for him? Hey, and he's supposedly the 'expert,' whom people who want to know turn to! Wake up, friends! When and where will all this nonsense end? The other magazines won't stop it—and the bodybuilders sure as hell won't because they're stuck; either you keep taking drugs and getting bigger and more cut, or you won't win contests or get an endorsement contract.

"Never in my life have I used any drug to build my body. Never! I wasn't born with the physique I built; I worked hard for it. Yet, I did it naturally. Sure, I didn't build it up to the size of today's drug–enhanced physiques, but I was after symmetry and proportion, and I achieved it in a package that allowed me to win the Mr. America and Mr. Universe titles, along with giving me a successful film career. Even today, at 71 years of age, I work on my ranch, work out and would be willing to bet that I could out–power walk many of those bloated muscle druggies 40 years my junior!

"To me, a bodybuilder is someone who not only builds his body naturally, but has functional, real–world muscle that can be used at any time, and will help the person perform any activity better.

"When it came to my body—the body you saw—and the condition I had, that was the body I had 24 hours a day, 365 days a year! I was not some bloated, out–of–shape, easily winded giant whose razor sharp physique could only stay that way for a few weeks before or after a contest.(I can just hear the directive from the magazine editor to the photographers, 'Hurry and snap those pictures before we lose him!').

"When Steve Blechman, Publisher and Editor—in–Chief of NATURAL MD, spoke to me about his vision for taking the sport back to its natural roots, I applauded him. For others in the industry have had the opportunity and have 'talked the talk,' but no one has had the guts to take a stand for what's right. Blechman has. And that is why, after all these years, I've decided to help the sport I love get back to its proper place. One of the ways I intend to do that is by writing a monthly column for NATURAL MD magazine.

"Something needs to be done now; we have no choice. For where there is no vision the people perish; and where there is no vision for the future of body-building, bodybuilding will perish.

"Many people may ask if there is another reason for me coming out of retirement to help save the sport. The answer is no, and I want to make one thing crystal clear: My passion for what I do has never been driven by money. I retired at the peak of my movie career, so that I could live life on my own terms.

"All my life, I have never answered to anyone and I'm not about to do it now. The only thing I can give you in the coming months—through the pages of this magazine—is honesty and the truth about building your body without drugs.

"I will teach you everything you will need to know to build the body you truly want. That is, to build it naturally and without any drugs. If you want to look like the other bodybuilders and want the latest drug information, then go to the other magazines. I'm only interested in talking about one thing: real bodybuilding. If that's what you want, then my friend, welcome home!"

TWELVE:

NOW IT'S MY TURN (Or Why I'm No Fan Of Arnold!)

"No one comes close to Reeves in stirring the heart by way of muscle and might, balance and striking feature, bearing and countenance."—Dave Draper, Champion Bodybuilder

STAY FIT(AND HOT)FOR LIFE

Why would I presume so audaciously to take up the torch—and cause—passed on so passionately and vehemently by Steve Reeves by advocating as he did drug–free bodybuilding and champion him so zealously above and beyond all other bodybuilder champions as the best and most perfect or ideal role model for any young person to emulate and follow so wisely? Because Steve built and perfected the most impeccable, incomparable, unique and one–of–a–kind classic physique the like of which the world had never before seen and will never see again. He did it naturally and exclusively by sheer hard–working desire, discipline and determination(what he called the *"3 Ds!"*). He set a standard of pure physical perfection which remains unmatched and unsurpassed to the present day—all without resort to bloated muscle tissue artificially induced by anabolic steroids or any other so–called growth–stimulating drugs or substances. He never followed anyone since he trained in his own distinctive but intensely strict style, striving to build his body in his own superlative and shape–specific way. And he proved beyond any and all question or doubt—pure and simple—that the aesthetic of sheer physical *BEAUTY* truly is superior to mere size or bulk amassed for their own sake.

Rick Wayne put it most eloquently for *All Natural Muscular Development* magazine(May 1997, Volume 34, Number 5, Page 205):

"I had come to realize the amazing body–parts that together totaled up to the world's most beautiful male body—those peerless shoulders, that minuscule waist, the dancer's hips, the uniquely connected Reeves pecs!—could not be duplicated. For indeed they were special gifts from the Creator. As for the face of Reeves that had given even the most macho of men good cause for pause—to say nothing of its varied effects on women!—the best one could do was try to put it out of one's mind, for fear it tempted one to blaspheme. Truly, Steve Reeves had always been one of a kind."

Others have echoed identical sentiments. "Thanks to his godlike appearance," David Chapman wrote in a brief biography, "Steve Reeves inspired an entire generation to take up weights and exercise so that they could look like he did. Of course, no one ever did look quite like him; Reeves had a kind of charisma and physical perfection that only comes along once in a generation. Being a god may have had its drawbacks, but we are grateful that he was there to inspire us all...No matter what he did, however, Reeves continued to have a great influence on hopeful musclemen. He showed a generation of young men the potentials of bodybuilding through his contest victories, his magazine articles, but most importantly through his appearance in movies. His handsome face, bold stage presence, and perfectly symmetrical physique destined the young muscleman for a role beyond the posing dais, and Steve Reeves did not disappoint those who saw in him a perfect spokesman for the burgeoning sport of bodybuilding. As a physique star and later as a popular film personality, Steve Reeves is living proof that a muscular build and a healthy lifestyle can translate into a successful career. His masculine good looks combined with his powerful physique provided a model for the young bodybuilders of an entire generation. To most of us, he still is god."

"It's doubtful that any bodybuilder in the history of the sport has had a broader mass influence and appeal than Steve Reeves," wrote John Little for

Flex magazine. "Certainly other champions have had larger muscles, been more ripped or more striated, but none have possessed the across-the-board appeal and perfection of form that reached its summit in the Reeves physique."(February 1993, Page 37).

"I believe it is because every muscle Reeves built on his body was purposeful," Little added, "enhanced or defined to bring a sense of proportion and symmetry to the eye with a sense of artistry and aesthetics that is sorely lacking from today's 'size for the sake of size' trainees...Also(and it's not a small point to be glossed over), Reeves built his body naturally; i.e., without steroids or other so–called 'bodybuilding drugs,' with the result that his body represented unadulterated human physiology—at its absolute zenith."(***Dynamic Muscle Building***, Page 6).

"The standards that he set for physical symmetry are a welcome relief from today's bodybuilders with bloated muscles and abdomens and with extreme vascularity," George Miller reflected for *Iron Game History*. "Steve had smooth, yet well–defined muscles with a slight vascularity that blended perfectly on a perfect frame. His photos and standards will survive long after today's current stars have faded."(December 2000, Volume 6, Number 4, Page 15).

Similarly, wrote Gene Mozee, "Steve Reeves introduced a whole new look to bodybuilding. His classical physique has never been equaled for sheer beauty and symmetry. If the great Michelangelo had Steve Reeves for a model, his statue of David would have undoubtedly looked remarkably like Steve Reeves as the perfect male physique...Steve Reeves was a superhero to his multi–millions of bodybuilding fans who became the ultimate superstar of action films in his era. No one before or since has ever been more

JOSEPH COVINO JR

acclaimed as the most perfectly developed man of all time."

"Just as there is feminine beauty there is masculine beauty," Ken "Leo" Rosa affirmed for *Iron Game History*, "and Steve Reeves represented its pinnacle in sharp contrast to the disgustingly ugly, pathologically grotesque steroid freaks of today."(December 2000, Volume 6, Number 4, Page 37).

"Even with today's vast choice of physiques," David Gentle wrote for *NaturalStrength.com*, "Steve Reeves, because of a combination of facial as well as physical beauty and symmetry, had, the most universally envied development in modern times...In spite of the passage of time—now some 50 years since he recorded his Mr. America victory and despite all the changes that have taken place in Bodybuilding's 'fashions'—Reeves has remained the pinnacle of perfection to millions of fans, with an aesthetic physique many still attempt to emulate. Real beauty is as has been said timeless as is good taste...History records Steve Reeves won the Mr. America, and all of five decades later, still remained one, if not the, most admired of all physique stars to grace the posing dais."(30 June 2000).

"The immortal Steve Reeves," wrote Dennis B. Weis, paying tribute to Steve for *Critical Bench.com*, "Reeves had the rugged handsome good looks, golden tan and magnificent incomparable physique of classic lines and proportions that were and continue to be appreciated not only by bodybuilders but the average man or woman, and that is a rarity, too! Reeves' impact of muscle aesthetics, impressive shape and symmetry, set a standard that still exists today. Broad champion shoulders, colossal wide back, tidy etched waist, trim hips, formidable thighs and diamond

184

shaped calves...Even today Reeves had what can be considered as perfect and socially accepted proportions. His rugged features, black hair and blue eyes left no doubt he was a movie star and his physique left no doubt he was Hercules."(16 October 2006).

So this humble and modest gentleman who honestly built without any sort of cheating whatever the most perfect male physique on the planet and raised his brave voice so passionately and tirelessly against the abuse and misuse of chemicals and drugs in natural bodybuilding—but who died so abruptly and prematurely in May 2000 at the age of 74 from a blood clot due to complications of lymphoma—must have known something of which he spoke! Steve Reeves felt that bodybuilding is supposed to be a jubilant celebration of fitness, health and longevity—not the sport's death knell!

That, in a nutshell, is why I'm no fan of Arnold Schwarzenegger or any of his bloated, mis–proportioned, unfit, unhealthy, substance–abusing, druggie bulk–builder ilk. Schwarzenegger, in fact, both embodies and personifies bogus bulk–building—epitomized in turn by three despicable and deplorable things: cigars, steroids and open–heart surgery. Not to mention worthless major motion picture films glorifying gratuitous slaughter and violence. To say nothing of outright outrageous discourtesy and disrespect: to my knowledge Schwarzenegger neither did Steve the simple courtesy nor paid him the simple respect this universally renowned bodybuilding pioneer so justly deserved by giving him a forthright and straightforward reply to Steve's impassioned plea for courageous collaboration against druggie bulk–building. Such derelict indifference and negligence amount to nothing but sheer craven cowardice! Presently, he's assumed the California governorship and could potentially run(figuratively speaking since bulk–builders can't run!)for even higher political office. Hopefully he'll speedily recover and re–consider since the very last thing either the state, nation or world–at–large needs is hypocritical AH–nold single–handedly ushering in yet another exploitative and oppressive Reagan–and–Bush–style era of neo–aristocratic/feudalistic domestic policy at home and neo–colonialist/hegemonic/imperialistic and warmongering foreign policy abroad.

In an interview with Roy Frumkes, editor of *The Perfect Vision* magazine, Steve forthrightly recounted his first meeting with the two–faced bulk–builder: "We were at Jack LaLanne's 65th birthday party, and Schwarzenegger came up to me and said, 'Steve, you've always been an idol of mine.' I looked him straight in the eye, half–smiling, and said, 'Don't give me that crap, Arnold. I read your book, and Reg Park was your idol.' He said, 'Well...only because I knew I couldn't look like you.'" Steve defeated Park for the Mr. Universe title in 1950.

Invariably, Steve portrayed honorable and noble movie characters who were valorous liberators of oppressed peoples. "He was no longer a desired commodity at the box office," John Fair concluded for *Iron Game History*, "not because he was a few years older or any less talented but because society had changed. The new realism of the 1970s, featuring gratuitous sex, foul language, drugs, vulgarity, and violence, flew directly against the values of the high–minded, clean–living Reeves. Steve personified qualities that were redolent of an earlier era...Reeves had epitomized the image of the perfect man and, perhaps more than any other major figure, represented the opposite of what bodybuilding and the motion picture industry was moving towards."(December 2000, Volume 6, Number 4, Page 33).

To his dying day, Steve tried so valiantly to liberate this country's impressionable and unsuspecting youth from the harmful ills of not only potentially fatal steroidal bulk–building but also detrimental training techniques and unhealthful synthetic supplements—all utterly ineffectual for the natural classic physique bodybuilder!

If the Arnold–like bulk–builder pretenders won't immediately *STOP* their atrocious misconduct and shameful mal–practices for the sake of their own fitness, health and longevity then they should immediately *STOP* corrupting our trustful youth with their misguided, misleading and misrepresented misinformation—or at the very least *HONESTLY* instruct them with the unvarnished *TRUTH* to empower them to make up their own minds and so they can make truly educated, enlightened and informed *FREE CHOICES* about which course to take!

"In many instances," Steve cautioned in his *PowerWalking* book, "our choice of conditioning activities is almost as counterproductive as our daily living habits. Everyone is constantly looking for a gimmick or a fad—the easy way. In response to this demand, everywhere you turn there is another new diet, exercise gimmick, or conditioning tool—anything to make us appear younger, thinner, sexier, bigger, smaller, or better. Few people seem satisfied with approaching their health in a scientific manner. No matter how bad the economy, Americans will find a way to afford the luxury of beauty. Much of this is done through advertising that ranges from classy to just plain ridiculous...Whatever the price, the general public seems willing to pay unlimited amounts of money to appear handsome or beautiful.

"People also seem to jump into any new activity promoting physical fitness as long as it appears that millions of others are doing the same and that the activity promises immediate results...As an outgrowth of this scenario, many people have been 'turned off' to exercise. This is extremely unfortunate."

"In many cases," Steve reiterated in his body-building book, "our choice of conditioning activities are almost as counterproductive as our daily living habits. Everyone seems to be looking for a gimmick or fad—the easy way. In response to this demand, everywhere you turn there is a new diet, exercise gimmick or conditioning tool—anything to make us look younger, thinner, sexier, bigger, smaller or better. Few people seem satisfied with approaching their health in a scientific manner. No matter how bad the economy, people will always find a way to afford the luxury of beauty. Truth be told, there is no quick fix. There is no miracle way to fitness or weight loss. But there are good and practical ways to achieve a firmer and more shapely body. These principles will not and have not changed."

WORDS OF PARTING
TO ASPIRING AND STRIVING YOUTH

Never let yourself be so habitually fooled and so easily deceived: every time you let yourself get sucked in by some amateur bulk–builder into practicing piss–poor weight–training techniques or ingesting harmful synthetic supplements, simply because he's perhaps won a couple "bodybuilding" trophies in amateur competitions perpetuating mis–proportioned physique standards—or worse, simply because you mis-perceive that he looks "big"—you're simply pandering to his puny ego but you're doing absolutely *NOTHING* whatever to advance or improve your own physique's muscular growth and development. *PROGRESS*—not stagnation and regression—is what *REAL* bodybuilding is all about. In short, *RESULTS*—concrete, real, tangible and visible *RESULTS*—are the name of the game! *RESULTS* motivate you to advance, develop, improve and *PROGRESS* even *FURTHER!* So long as you lick the feet of any amateur bulk–builder for all the *WRONG REASONS*(he's "big" and he's won some amateur trophies)you only puff up his puny ego at the precious expense of your own physique's muscular growth and development! It's just that plain and simple. So *WISE UP!* Get *SMART* and *HABITUATE* yourself to *TRUE FITNESS, HEALTH AND LONGEVITY* instead! Don't inflict upon yourself an *OUT–OF–SHAPE, SHORT–WINDED, STATIC AND UNFUNCTIONAL PHYSIQUE* that never, ever changes much less improves or progresses! That's neither more nor less than *INEFFECTUAL MOVEMENT WITHOUT RESULT!* In short, that's physique–*IMPOTENCE!*

Now there's absolutely nothing whatever wrong with picking and choosing ideal role models to emulate and follow presuming they're truly admirable and exemplary—meaning that they're preferably *NATURAL AND WORLD–CLASS!* In both of these respects Steve Reeves was *PEERLESS!* "Steve Reeves," wrote Preston Rendell, Mr. USA(Natural)in a letter of tribute for *Muscle Mag International*(October 2000), "was, is and always will be Hercules. He was put on the Earth to inspire youths to take up bodybuilding, fitness and the disciplined lifestyle that goes with them." As Dave Ferrier put it in his "Tombstone Tribute" for *WildestWesterns.com*, "Mr. Reeves was certainly a wholesome role model for his generation and those to come." And Lou Ravelle for *NaturalStrength.com*, "I think he must have provided more inspiration for beginners than any other, before or since. Unforgettable, impeccable and irreplaceable. He had a combination of grace, power and line, which has never been matched, and never will be."(30 June 2000). "There will always be individuals so immersed in negativity that they project it onto everyone around them," Ken "Leo" Rosa pointed out for *Iron Game History*. "They bemoan and criticize the fact that Steve could not match(so–and–so's)strength...The reality is that he didn't have to do that. All he had to do was to be what he was. An inspiration. An icon. One of the greatest natural bodybuilders of all time. Natural."(December 2000, Volume 6, Number 4, Page 37).

So long as you persist in licking the feet of some amateur bulk–builder like a lapdog by practicing his piss–poor weight–training techniques and ingesting his harmful synthetic supplements you assure yourself of only one thing for sure: ***SUREFIRE FAILURE! AND NOT ONE INFINITESIMAL IOTA OF DEVELOPMENT OR IMPROVEMENT IN YOUR PHYSIQUE!***

"I think the poor form is the result of trying to use too much weight," Steve cautioned youth directly, "or by watching some other guy working out who was using poor form and then copying him. Let's say you're sixteen or eighteen years old and the guy you're watching train is 25–years–old and he has big arms and big lats—you might automatically think that what he's doing must be the right way. However, it may have taken him 10 years to get those big arms and lats, when it would have taken him only two years if he did the exercise correctly."(*Dynamic Muscle Building*, Page 41).

CHECKLIST
FOR TRUE FITNESS, HEALTH
AND LONGEVITY
(Or Use Your HEAD—that is, your LOGIC, REASON AND COMMON SENSE!)

Stop kidding yourself, take off the *BLINDERS* and take a good, hard *LOOK* at that over–bloated bulk–builder you're so prone to lick the feet of like a lapdog and *THINK!* Honestly answer for yourself some few simple questions to *MAKE UP YOUR OWN MIND* and *DECIDE DEFINITELY FOR YOURSELF* whether it's worth your time and effort to pander to his equally over–bloated ego at the precious expense of your own physique's muscular growth and development:

•**DO YOU HONESTLY WANT TO LOOK LIKE HE DOES?** Do you honestly want to build a freakish, over–bloated and grotesque physique with overdeveloped trapezius and oblique muscles with everything else mis–proportioned? Because if you emulate his piss–poor training techniques and ingest his harmful synthetic supplements—and if your muscle fibers remotely match his—you stand some small chance of starting to look like him. In all likelihood, though, you'll never, ever look anything like him(because your muscle fibers are likely nothing like his)and you'll merely labor senselessly and wastefully in vain! Since his puny ego won't let him admit the truth to you it's your call.

•**DO YOU HONESTLY WANT TO SACRIFICE YOUR PHYSIQUE'S NATURALLY PROPORTIONATE, SYMMETRICAL AND PLEASING LOOK AS WELL AS YOUR REAL–WORLD**

FUNCTIONAL ABILITY? Because if you do emulate his piss–poor training techniques and ingest his harmful synthetic supplements then you most certainly will sacrifice everything about your physique that's aesthetically pleasant and pleasing!

•**DO YOU HONESTLY WANT TO BUILD A PHYSIQUE WITH ALL STYLE AND NO SUBSTANCE?** No matter how "big" or how "strong" an over–bloated physique gets it's still *FUNCTIONALLY USELESS*—that is, *PHYSIQUE–IMPOTENT!*—without the other *CRUCIAL FUNCTIONS OF TOTAL FITNESS, HEALTH AND LONGEVITY: AEROBIC CAPACITY AND MUSCULAR FLEXIBILITY!*

•**DO YOU HONESTLY WANT TO BUILD YOUR PHYSIQUE BY CHEATING?** Because that's what ingesting his synthetic chemicals, drugs, hormones and similar supplements amounts to.

•**DOES HE HONESTLY LOOK FAT, SICKLY AND OUT–OF–SHAPE CLOTHED OR DRESSED?** Examine his *OVER–BLOATED FACE CLOSELY*—a *PUFFY(SWOLLEN)FACE* with obscurely defined cheekbones and jaw–line and saggy jowls is indeed a *DEAD GIVEAWAY* for an unfit, unhealthy and untrained human being—no matter how "muscular" his physique may be!

•**DOES HE GET SHORT–WINDED AT PRACTICING THE LEAST BIT OF AEROBIC EXERCISE? DOES HE PLOP HIMSELF DOWN ON A BENCH OUT–OF–BREATH IN–BETWEEN SETS OF WEIGHTS?** If he does that should tell you *SOMETHING!*

•**DOES HE LOOK LIKE THE TRAINING TECHNIQUES AND SYNTHETIC SUPPLEMENTS HE ADVOCATES WORK FOR HIM?** If so then that's all well and good *FOR HIM!* If not, then you must *LOGICALLY AND RATIONALLY CONSIDER THE SOURCE!* In the end you must *USE YOUR COMMON SENSE* and ask the most crucial question: will what he advocates *WORK FOR YOU? WHY OR WHY NOT? IF YOU DON'T KNOW THEN FIND OUT!*

•**DOES HE PROFUSELY HARP UPON, "NO PAIN, NO GAIN," AND THEN ONCE YOU PRACTICE HIS PISS–POOR TRAINING TECHNIQUES THAT'S PRECISELY WHAT YOU FEEL: PAIN?** Wake up! If you're suffering hurtful *PAIN* that's aching your joints at the ankles, elbows, hips, knees, lower back, shoulders, wrists or anyplace else in your body then you're training *INCORRECTLY* and should immediately *STOP* training that way! If *COMMON SENSE* doesn't kick in then permanently damaged joints, ligaments or tendons eventually will!

•**DO YOU ACTUALLY SEE ANY CONCRETE, REAL, TANGIBLE AND VISIBLE RESULTS IN AT LEAST ONE MONTH'S TIME FROM EMULATING OR FOLLOWING WHATEVER HE ADVOCATES?** Naturally, that presumes you've already been *SUCKED IN* to emulating or following whatever he advocates. If you train and work out day after day, week after week, month after month, year after year and your physique *STAYS UTTERLY STATIC AND UNCHANGING* then I don't care whether the current "Mr. Olympia" himself is training you: whatever he's trying to sell you *WILL NOT WORK FOR YOU AND LIKELY NEVER WILL! COMMON SENSE MUST FINALLY KICK IN SOONER OR LATER AND TELL YOU THAT THERE MUST BE ANOTHER AND BETTER WAY!* And if that's the case for you then I challenge you to try Steve's way devotedly for just one month to achieve guaranteed results!

Real muscular growth and development result from correct(often arduous)training, correct diet(getting your essential nutrients from balanced, healthful and wholesome food!)along with plenty of rest and recuperation. It never comes out of practicing piss–poor training techniques or ingesting harmful synthetic supplements—much less licking the feet of an amateur bulk–builder like a lapdog! Building a classic physique naturally results from neither more nor less than hard work and working out! It all boils down to whether you're willing to do the work—correctly!

"Quit looking for miracles in a pill, packet or powder," Steve advised for *All Natural Muscular Development* magazine. "At best, they may only help. Get your body in the gym and under the iron and keep it there for as long as it takes for you to have the body you want. That's the way you build it and keep it. It's always been like that and it will always be like that!"(December 1997, Volume 34, Number 12, Page 130).

If I have saved any single one of you from falling prey to the bane of bulk–building then writing this book will have proved well worth the effort!

So what are just sitting there reading this for? Get yourself into your gym and get to **WORK!**

AFTERWORD:
A SUPERIOR AND SUPERLATIVE PAST

"Steve Reeves was 'IT.' There are many stars but he was a supernova who, in bodybuilding terms, transcended all those before him and since. From head to foot Steve Reeves was superlative."—Malcolm Whyatt, Oscar Heidenstam Foundation Archivist and Historian

Plenty of people most mistakenly think that whatever's past—including the icons, ideals and idols of yesteryear—is automatically and necessarily passé, and even its most celebrated and illustrious heroes old–fashioned, out–of–date and out–of–style. So often they're outright overlooked and unjustly forgotten as has–been relics of ancient history.

"Likewise," wrote Ken O'Neill in an article for *Dolfzine Online Fitness* titled, ***Bodybuilding's Mythic Hero: Reclaiming the Image***, "Steve Reeves, upon passing, fared only slightly better, no doubt due to his legacy of having portrayed Hercules in films. Steve Reeves' death should have been covered heavily by the mainstream media. For a few short years, besides having won the Mr. Universe and other major bodybuilding titles, he was a major film star.

"People who participate in bodybuilding form a culture whether they know it or not. And the values of that culture are reflected in the recognition that people like...Reeves received in their lives for the ways they struggled and all they achieved. These men fulfilled the mythic image of the successful bodybuilder while they were alive, but for some reason, seem to have been relegated to a dusty shelf when it comes to being remembered today...

"The mythology of bodybuilding appears to be crumbling, as its finest heroes ride off into the sunset, too often forgotten...Reeves showed today's bodybuilders what human potential, left to natural devices, can accomplish."

Why then should Steve Reeves be permanently recognized and remembered not only today but for all time to come?

"There is good reason to believe that Reeves

should actually be called the first bodybuilder," wrote O'Neill.

"He trained for size, shape and proportion rather than for strength—one of the main differences between bodybuilding and other forms of weight training...Reeves should be credited with setting the standard for pure bodybuilding concerned with developing the optimal masculine physique based on an aesthetic standard which inspired several decades of bodybuilders...

"Perhaps letting the old heroes of bodybuilding die quietly serves some purpose, the result of which is selective amnesia. Forgetting about how the greats of the past did it, after all, means not having to admit to not being able to live up to that image...

"Tomorrow's bodybuilders face a really tough challenge. Living up to the mythic image created by the great bodybuilding heroes of the past and competing with their advancements will take a lot of working out. Those of us who continue to believe that bodybuilding is a way to being awake and promoting good health certainly hope they will give it a try."

In more blunt terms, the so-called "champions" of the supposedly superior contemporary "new school" of bodybuilding readily dismiss the natural champions of the classical "old school" of bodybuilding to conveniently avoid admitting their inability to excel except by taking the easiest and quickest route: cheating rather than exerting!

"People who are younger do often dismiss the past as passé without realizing that some of the basic truths are not changed by time or fads," astutely wrote Deborah Engelhorn–Reeves–Stewart, Steve's wife. "Taking care of your body by common sense and educated choices is not old–fashioned—it's just harder and therefore rarer."

I'll conclude directly by rebutting the most absurd and idiotic commentary encountered yet concerning Steve Reeves.

"Frankly," wrote Clarence Bass at his *Ripped* website, "I've never been very interested in Steve Reeves...The fact that his body responded to training so miraculously suggested to me that his methods had little or no relevance to other people. Plus, the fact that he gave up serious training early in life made me even less interested in him...I was probably correct about his training methods, but I now realize that Steve Reeves had something more important to offer. He was, of course, an inspiration to many bodybuilders. It made little difference that any attempt to imitate him was probably folly."

"That's an amazing thing," Steve himself unknowingly concurred with Bass on at least one salient point in his unrelated interview with Roy Frumkes. "My body responds so well to exercise, and it keeps it so long, that I didn't have to(work out a lot). I didn't take any steroids, they didn't exist at that time. It was just easy for me to get in shape and to stay in shape."

Steve, Les Stockton likewise confirmed for *Iron Game History*, "had a body that easily and quickly responded to weight training."(December 2000, Volume 6, Number 4, Page 26).

To stupidly suggest that Steve's methods and techniques hold little or no "relevance" for "other people" simply because Steve's body "responded" so superbly and so supremely to his own training is asinine and silly. His body's stupendous response to his own training, quite the contrary, is precisely the primary reason why Steve's methods and techniques prove beyond any and all doubt to be the most relevant—not to mention the most effective and efficient—for anyone and everyone striving to attain the best and most results in the least time. Following Steve Reeves is "probably folly?" Far from it! Failing to follow Steve Reeves is more likely the profoundest and worst folly!

Without fail, suffice it to say, I'd aspire to emulate Steve Reeves before I'd ever even think about taking after self–styled "champion bodybuilder," Clarence Bass, frankly. Forget for the time being his bald–as–an–egg head together with his withered and wrinkled face. In spite of his mediocre and moderately muscular physique he doubtless looks old beyond his years. Relative to Reeves, Bass isn't fit to hold a proverbial candle to the perfect proportion and symmetry belonging to the most magnificent natural classic physique the world has ever witnessed!

In the same belittling breath though—in all fairness—Bass rightfully praised Steve for all the right reasons.

"Perhaps the handsomest and certainly one of the best built men of his era," Bass seemed to grudgingly eulogize Steve, "Reeves motivated many people to start training, and to continue serious training long after he stopped. But Reeves was more than a bodybuilding icon. With all his natural gifts and fame, he remained a humble man. He led a clean, dignified and scandal–free life. To my way of thinking, that makes his life worth remembering, especially in this day and age of fallen idols and crumbling mores."

John Fair eulogized Steve for *Iron Game History* with exactly identical sentiments: "He was not only one of the handsomest and best built men of his era, but he led a clean, dignified, and scandal–free life."(December 2000, Volume 6, Number 4, Page 28).

Perhaps one plagiarized the other. Or perhaps one is a pen–name for the other, for all I know or care, though Fair similarly observed: "His body responded easily to weight training in size, strength, and proportion."(Page 29).

Well, Steve certainly motivated me to train despite the fact that we never even met. I for one would never—in the words of Clarence Bass—"attempt to imitate" or pattern my own physique after anyone else, much less Clarence Bass, frankly. I haven't. I wouldn't. I won't.

"Take it from one who knows—me," Steve exhorted us all. "If you are serious about a complete body development, you can—by persistence, patience, intelligent effort and a state of mind which says, 'I WILL,' instead of 'I hope to,' improve your physique to a point where it is practically flawless."(***Dynamic Muscle Building***, Page 97). Those were wise words I took to heart.

Building a natural classic physique you're perfectly pleased with and proud of is what it's all about. And to my way of thinking, Steve's training methods and techniques—and Steve's alone—have worked wonders for me and my own natural classic physique on the passing of my fiftieth birthday....and beyond!

For that, my appreciation and gratitude for Steve Reeves and his ever relevant training is eternal and everlasting—as, in a manner of speaking, ***"IMMENSE AND IMMORTAL WERE THE DEEDS OF HERCULES!"***

And indeed, concluded Oscar Heidenstam Foundation Archivist and Historian, Malcolm Whyatt, for *Iron Game History*, "Steve Reeves is a pyramid among the immortals."(December 2000, Volume 6, Number 4, Page 38).

If you really enjoyed reading this book then kindly write and post a favorable reader review for it at its pages at both *Amazon.com* **and** *Barnes and Noble.com.* **THANK YOU!!**

APPENDIX I

JOSEPH COVINO JR'S STATS

Birth-date: 24 January 1954
Height: 6–foot–2-inches
Weight: 210 pounds(small bones)
Shoulder Breadth: 18 inches
Chest: 44 inches
Waist: 34 inches
Hips: 38 inches
Biceps: 16 inches
Thigh: 24 inches
Calf: 16 inches

Contact JOSEPH COVINO JR, CFT:
josephcovinojr@gmail.com

Nationally Recognized Fitness Trainer Certifications

American Council On Exercise(ACE)
International Sports Sciences Association(ISSA)
National Academy of Sports Medicine(NASM)
National Council On Strength And Fitness(NCSF)
National Federation of Personal Trainers(NFPT)
National Strength
And Conditioning Association(NSCA)

APPENDIX II

A CAUTIONARY WARNING
TO PARENTS OF YMCA KIDS

Every gym, commercial and non–profit alike, most likely has its resident bulk–builder camp, clique or contingent. When it comes to the bulk–builder band operating out of your local YMCA, typically with the tacit approval and blessing of even the ruling echelons of Y administrations, what parents don't know(but ought to find out about)might potentially hurt, injure or otherwise permanently cripple or disable their imperiled posterity. What I've personally observed over a period spanning several years at the so–called "downtown" Berkeley YMCA poses an outright terrifying case–in–point. An apparently indifferent administration has given its own resident bulk–builder free reign to run rampant teaching unsuspecting youth who know no better downright detrimental if not dangerous weight–training habits(outlined in detail in Chapter Three). This particular bulk–builder is permitted to operate carte blanche, presumably due to that stand–by alibi: he's "big" and he's won some amateur bulk–building trophies. Well, it should take no rocket scientist to figure out the fallacy and flaw of such misguided presumption—especially once you witness the persistent spectacle of those gullible and sheepish young dupes repeatedly plopping themselves down on benches, immediately following their dubious exercises, groping in conspicuous pain their connective joints(like elbows, shoulders and wrists)time after time, time and time again! In word both spoken and written I've brought the matter to the notice of that particular Y's deliberately deaf, dumb and blind administration. In rebuttal all I've gotten is what I term the stupidly silent but witlessly wagging head of *DENIAL*.

Sample observations:

•Upright Row(barbell): with a wide, wrist–stressing grip, jerking the barbell up to the chin and dropping it, repeatedly, without pause or negative rep resistance.

•Standing–Front–Raise(barbell): with a straight–arm grip, swinging the barbell up and down for momentum, using lower–back leverage, without pause or negative rep resistance.

•Bent–Over Lateral Raise(dumbbells): bent–over at only a 45–degree angle jerking and swinging up the dumbbells with bent elbows for momentum and dropping the dumbbells without pause or negative rep resistance.

•Supine Bench Press(barbell): assisted reps of extremely excessive weight beneath which the unsuspecting dupe could not even conceivably be expected to press on their own.

•Supine Pullover(dumbbell): with upper torso sideways across a flat bench, upper back against the bench, stressed head raised, stressed neck, stressed lower back hanging down, stressed knees bent.

•One–Arm Row(dumbbell): with a torque torso jerking up excessively heavy weight to the shoulder for momentum and dropping it without pause or negative rep resistance.

•Low–Pulley Row(cable row machine): jerking excessively heavy weight and heaving the whole body back and forth in a seesaw motion for momentum without pause or negative rep resistance

•Standing Curl(barbell): swinging excessively heavy weight up and down for momentum without pause or negative rep resistance, elbows flared—out from the body, leaning backward with the upper back and shoulders for leverage.

•Seated Scott Bench Curl(dumbbell): jerking the weight up and down, elbows flared—out, half—way movements without pause or negative rep resistance, leaning back with upper back and shoulders for leverage.

•Alternate Curl(dumbbells): alternately bouncing and swinging up one excessively heavy dumbbell in one hand from the hip for momentum(without pause or negative rep resistance)while dropping down the second dumbbell in the other with elbows flared—out for leverage.

•Triceps Press—down(high pulley bar): frenetic jerk—down movements for momentum without pause or negative rep resistance, elbows flared—out, upper back and shoulders bowed over for leverage.

•French Press—Behind—Neck(dumbbell): half—way, jerk-up—and—drop movements for momentum without pause or negative rep resistance.

•Bent—Over Triceps Extension(dumbbell): frenetic, jerk—back—and—up movements without pause or negative rep resistance.

•Standing Calf Raises(leg—press machine): bouncing up and down on the balls of the feet with bent knees with half—way movements for momentum.

•Curl—Up and Sit—Up: jerking up the upper body and bouncing up and down for momentum.

•Knee—Up(vertical station): swinging straight legs together up and down for momentum.

"Never," cautions the encyclopedic *Personal Trainer Manual*(1997)by the **American Council on Exercise**, "have children perform single maximal lifts, sudden explosive movements or try to compete with other children."(Page 345).

In the spirit of truth and fair play, then, Berkeley YMCA VP/Executive Director, Fran Gallati, is herein invited to rebut and refute the content of this section(At print time Gallati had still ignored the written invitation sent months before publication).

Postscript

In his powerfully pandering "fluff" piece for *North Gate News Online* titled "Fitness Experts: Kids Should Grow Up Before Bulking Up"(11 November 2003), Peter Orsi, regurgitating gratuitous quotes from dubious conformist sources(parroting almost identical themes without any varied confutation or contradiction whatever)for the UC Berkeley Graduate School of Journalism—which apparently perpetuates the stenographer's transcript–style(rather than an analytical or even interpretative–style)of "reporting"—predictably puffed up the selfsame already over–bloated amateur bulk-builder: "As a 12–time bodybuilding contest champion, Berkeley YMCA fitness instructor(named)knows a thing or two about pumping iron."

Wrong. That's exactly the sort of misguided and misinformed presumption that misleads countless youth to practice so habitually yet so witlessly so many ineffectual and detrimental if not outright hurtful weight–training techniques. He's "big"("Broad–shouldered, with hulking biceps," Orsi puffed)and he's won some amateur contest trophies, so he must automatically and necessarily know what he's talking about—or so goes the unduly irrational line of ill-logic!

Big biceps, perhaps. Broad shoulders—most definitely not. In point of fact he displayed the mis–proportioned round–shouldered syndrome suffered by most contemporary bulk–builders of his ilk afflicted with the turtle–necked deformity attributable to the over–developed trapezius muscle at the base of the neck.

That's neither here nor there really: contemporary(and faulty) "bodybuilding" competition standards habitually patronize, promote and perpetuate bulk over balanced proportion and symmetry in physique development—bestowing contest trophies not for the best developed and most beautiful but rather just the biggest and bulkiest physiques.

That's beside the point really: your gym's resident bulk–builder might be blessed with exceptionally gifted genetics and muscle–fiber response to exercise—particularly weight–training(even if slipshod and sloppy). It might've taken him way more years than necessary to bloat up those big, bulky biceps had he not neglected to weight–train beneficially, correctly and most efficiently in perfect form and strict style for the most results in the least time! Besides that, his fitness level is likely more cosmetic than concrete if he's all form(all bulk)and no function(all anaerobic and no aerobic capacity to speak of).

Never let yourself get suckered so stupidly into swallowing that propagandistic "bigger–is–better" bait–trap of deficient if not outright detrimental weight–training techniques! What's "right" and what seemingly works for that big, bad bulk–builder may be woefully wrong and never, ever work for you(befitting your natural height and bone structure)!

So get wise and get the message: train for real results—not a lot of **TALK** and **WISHFUL THINK-ING!**

APPENDIX III

PICKING A "PERSONAL TRAINER"

In her weekly "Fit Smart" column for *USA Weekend* contributing editor, Stephanie Oakes, advised: "Do not hire a trainer on the basis of his looks. Just because a trainer has a great physique does not mean he has the necessary experience or knowledge."(14-16 February, 2003).

Well, he must've had the "necessary experience or knowledge" to build that "great physique" for himself if indeed it's that "great" at all. Physique quality naturally varies by both perception and standard—either of which might be deeply distorted.

So I'd qualify that advice: employ what I prefer to term a *fitness* trainer "on the basis of his looks" if he or she possesses a physique which *you* would personally aspire to build for yourself.

Jill Kinney, owner of *Club One* commercial(profiteering)fitness centers in the San Francisco Bay Area, likewise advised potential fitness clients in an interview with the *San Francisco Chronicle* to employ only those fitness trainers "certified" by one of three arbitrary certifying associations which test candidates in guidebook–type "knowledge."

"Would you go to a physician who wasn't certified, or who hadn't passed his or her board exams?" Kinney asked rhetorically in her lame attempt to sound profound. "You're dedicating your body to someone. It's in your best interest to make sure they know what they're talking about."(16 March 2003).

"'How do I look like Barbie?' I've heard some women ask," *San Francisco Bay Club* certified fitness instructor and director of fitness operations, Melissa

Kitz, asked rhetorically in her equally lame attempt to sound profound in her interview with the *San Francisco Chronicle.* "You can't. She's not reality."(24 August 2003)

Well, Barbie may not be "reality," but a truly conscientious and client–concerned fitness "instructor" could proselytize more positively by heartening such women that they can indeed with correct training and nutrition look **BETTER** than Barbie—a scrawny, mis–proportioned, inanimate, miniature kewpie doll, after all!

Personally, I prefer my fitness trainer to be an expert and professional practitioner rather than some amateur, armchair, handbook–reading theorist. Steve Reeves was a master practitioner par excellence!

Putting your misplaced trust in some "certified" fitness trainer simply because they're "certified" falsely presumes that the source of their supposed "education and examination"—their various personal trainer manuals—is well–founded and valid. It often isn't. So "certification" scarcely qualifies them to automatically and necessarily "know what they're talking about."

As for physicians, so–called, they must rate high as being among the least fit and healthy people inhabiting the planet—despite their sometimes auto mechanical–style advances in surgery! Besides, these pill–pushing quacks ply their professional trade mostly by peddling prescription drugs—the last thing you want to resort to in building a classic physique the natural way!

"There's a wonderful anabolic and health promoting component to gelatin—or at least I found that to be the case," Steve once expounded, recounting his own experience with physicians. "I recall some years ago that I was diagnosed with a duodenal ulcer. I'm not big on hospitals, so their advice to me was to stay home—in bed—and follow a bland diet. I'm a very intuitive individual and I think my intuition cured me of the ulcer—and here's how: I had this incredible craving for Jell-O. I would eat bowls of the stuff during this period and I would thicken it with plain gelatin every day. Within two months, the symptoms of the duodenal ulcer had disappeared. And when I went back for X–rays the doctors told me that not only was I completely cured, but there was no sign of scar tissue, either. I believe to this day that the pure protein within the gelatin helped to cure me. I had a need for it and for its pure protein. I believe instinct and intuition can sometimes show you the way to better health."

"I think again intuition helped me," Steve told Armand Tanny in an interview. "I was able to cure myself in my own way. You see, I had a terrible craving for Jell–O and so I ate bowls of it, thickened with plain Knox gelatin every day. Within two months, the symptoms had disappeared. Several months later, out of curiosity, I went back for X–rays, and the doctors told me that not only was I completely cured, that there was no sign of scarring. I strongly believe to this day that the gelatin cured me. I had a need for it and for its pure protein...I believe instinct and intuition can show you the way. It is more than believing. I didn't consciously think gelatin was going to cure me. It was just something I felt I had to have. I guess it was nature's way of telling me 'there's your cure.'"(Chris LeClaire, Page 234).

So far as I know, Steve Reeves was never "certified" as a fitness trainer. What I do know is that this exceptional and extraordinary bodybuilding champion and fitness practitioner possessed more "necessary experience or knowledge" than all the world's certification boards, manuals and personal trainers combined! You can confidently "dedicate your body" to that!

APPENDIX IV

GENETIC GROUNDS TO REFRAIN FROM BULK–BUILDING

If sound reason, logic and common sense still aren't enough to deter you from practicing the bane of bulk–building even after you've frittered away hours, days, weeks, months and even years following some bulk–builder around your gym like a lapdog for absolutely no other rational reason whatever except that he's "big" or he's won some amateur contest trophies then sensibly consider the genetic grounds for trying not only a different but better way to build and develop your physique. Then get a good grip and let it finally *SINK IN: BULK–BUILDING WON'T WORK FOR YOU!*

•**Limb Length**. People with shorter limbs generally may lift more weight resistance(heavier poundage)than people with longer limbs since favorable leverage factors enhance their effective force(strength) output. So shorter–limbed people are at a definite advantage strength–wise.

•**Muscle Length**. Connective tissue called tendons attach muscles to bones. Some people have long muscles with short tendon attachments relative to their bone length. Others have short muscles with long tendon attachments relative to their bone length. Those with relatively longer muscles have greater potential for developing size and strength than those with relatively shorter muscles.

•**Tendon Insertion**. That point of tendon insertion is another factor that affects effective muscle strength. With a biceps tendon that attaches to the forearm farther from the elbow joint there's a biomechanical advantage which enables the lifting of more weight resistance in elbow–flexing exercises.

•**Muscle Fiber Type**. Most people possess a relatively even combination of fast–twitch and slow–twitch fibers in most of their skeletal muscles. Some people inherit a higher percentage of fast–twitch muscle fibers which enhances their performance potential for power activities(like sprinting). Others inherit a higher percentage of slow–twitch muscle fibers which enhances their performance potential for endurance exercise(like long–distance running). Both muscle fiber types respond positively to progressive strength resistance training. Fast–twitch muscle fibers though experience greater gains in both size and strength(hypertrophy). So people possessing a preponderance of fast–twitch muscle fibers might attain better results from their strength-training regimens.

APPENDIX V

FITNESS FRAUDS

PROTEIN BARS. I hate to burst your protein bar addiction bubble, but these ultra–convenient, user–friendly, and over–hyped "protein" bars are one of the worst and most atrocious fitness frauds ever perpetrated against the unsuspecting public. Why? Your typical "high–protein" bar maxes out at 20–22 grams of **QUALITY**, muscle–building protein, which is all that can be stuffed into the bar due to restrictions in the manufacturing process. Yet, some bars claim to contain 30–plus grams of protein by adding inferior, low–grade, barely–functioning protein. Then comes the claim that protein bars are better because they cater to the low–or–no–carb craze. That's crazy, all right, since *complex*(good)carbohydrates—those low–glycemic–value carbohydrates—are absolutely beneficial. In their place is substituted *glycerin*(neither a fat, protein, or carbohydrate)to dilute the bar so it doesn't taste detrimental from too much protein; *glycerin* adds both grams and calories to the bars. Worse still, for increased shelf life protein bars add substantial fat of the artery–blocking variety due to their high cholesterol content: partially–hydrogenated vegetable oils—otherwise notoriously known as trans–fats! You might well call these nasty things heart–stopper bars! Avoid them like the plague.

BOTIQUE FITNESS STUDIOS. *"Instead of working out in cavernous multi–purpose gyms,"* San Francisco Chronicle groupie, Mandy Behbehani, wrote "freelance," no less, in her puff–piece titled, *"Getting Into The Botique Fitness Zone"*(Sunday,

5 February 2017), *"more than 54 million exercise buffs are gathering these days for intense, personalized sessions in small, stylish, theme–oriented venues that often offer a single discipline sport like cycling."*

Well, isn't that all just so chic and modish?

"The trend covers rigorous cross–training outfits like CrossFit...and franchise chains like Orange Theory Fitness, where the workout focuses on intervals of cardiovascular and strength training with performance tracking. The trend also takes in studios that specialize in one or two sports like bike riding or barre," Behbehani wrote.

Reputedly, this so–called "trend" started in Manhattan(where else?), and ever uncreative, unimaginative and unoriginal San Francisco has to jump on the botique fitness studio bandwagon and play copycat!

Behbehani rambles on to puff one unmentionable "studio" that supposedly *"offers a strenuous, no–frills, heart–pumping circuit workout...intense sweat sessions...performed fast....These include planks, squat jumps, burpees and sit–ups."*

Well, that's the fast–track to **NOWHERE** when it comes to true health and fitness, longevity, and most importantly, weight control. It's likewise the fast–track to fleecing your pocketbook and wallet!

At another unmentionable "studio": *"Exercisers wear heart monitors that broadcast their heart rate and calories burned...on overhead screens...The arduous, 55–minute workout combines cardio on treadmills and rowers with push–ups, planks, crunches, free weights and more."*

Oh, and **MORE!** This puff–piece amounted *more* to a glorified advertisement than special–interest article–and an exceptionally deceptive advertisement, at that!

And yet another unmentionable "studio," according to publicist, Behbehani: *"runs three types of 40–minute classes: yoga, cycle…and sculpt, which takes a traditional classic pilates reformer workout and melds it with intense aerobic exercise."*

These con–jobbing charlatans gull their gullible, deluded dupes into believing that all that frenetic, stop–and–go, and vacuous activity is beneficial simply because it gets people winded and out of breath in a short time, lulling them into a false sense of complacency that they've vigorously "worked out." Run in place energetically for a hundred count and you'll attain the exact same breathless sensation. And that's just your **WARM–UP!**

Truth be told, these sorts of frenetic activities might improve your physical speed and power—marginally. But they'll do next to **NOTHING** to help develop, improve or change your body composition, much less help you to burn your body's fat stores to lose weight. One is done through correct weight–training, the other through bouts of continuous, steady–state aerobic exercise!

This is the undiluted truth and reality of the matter—not the false, deceptive and misleading **MAKE–BELIEVE** of the so–called "botique studio."

"EXPERT" GURUS. In yet another *San Francisco Chronicle* puff–piece, by Carolyne Zinko and Tony Bravo, titled, *"Secrets of aging well: Experts' advice on putting your best face(and body)forward,"* aka, *"How to look your absolute best—at any age"*(Sunday, 20 May 2018), a short–and–busty–and–*chunky* older gal named **Shari Shryock**, "fitness and wellness trainer," was a featured "expert." She's billed as "an award–winning competitive bodybuilder and fitness coach with 30 years in the personal training business." Ever hear of her? Nor have I.

"Looking your age in 2018 to me is not looking your age in 2018," Shryock was quoted as saying. "It's looking younger than your age, and most of the people I work with really want to look a bit younger than their natural ages…and I'm an example of what my business is about. I'm older(66)than most of the people I see, and they say, 'Well, if you can look like that'…"

Not intending to sound unkind, but all I have to say is: look this lady up and see for yourself what she looks like "for her age." And that's all I'll say, except to add like Steve: if whatever this person preaches so obviously hasn't worked for her, it's not about to **EVER WORK FOR YOU!** Enough said! So much for the over–hyped "experts."

WITLESS COLUMNISTS. Ignore the **IGNORANT**, uninformed, or worse, mis–informed in gyms, especially if they write self–indulgent columns in abysmal ad rags like the *San Francisco Chronicle.*

In her column titled, *"**Getting all worked up while working out**,"*(Friday, 13 September 2019), Vanessa Hua, along with Caille Millner the *Chron*'s Co–Whiner–Victim–in–Chief, bellyached like a crybaby:

"I thought about all the bad behavior, intentional or not, that I've witnessed over the years at gyms. Exercise is supposed to relieve stress, improve health and enhance your sense of well–being, yet I've also seen how tempers can flare between adults sharing space and equipment."

Naturally, and most conveniently, Hua excludes her own little self from exhibiting or practicing any "bad behavior." Of course, she's a perfect little angel when she goes to the gym to prejudge her fellow exercisers! Right off, though, she displays a wholesale ignorance of what exercise is really all about when she refers to it in such generic terms, accounting for why her own runty stature stays static and unchanging in spite of any "exercise" she pretends to perform.

To be truly effective, you see, exercise must always aspire after *SPECIFIC*(not general)goals and purposes: combining aerobic and anaerobic conditioning to a balanced degree, for example—building a strong muscular look and muscular endurance together with a high degree of cardiopulmonary fitness!

Citing some ridiculously silly female–centric "study," Hua, resumes her girly–gurl bellyaching:

"Women detailed how men consumed more space at the gym, in terms of the exercise they performed, grunting and groaning as they lifted heavy weights, or hogging equipment. They tried to stay out of the way of men, rushing to finish their workouts, tiptoeing and apologizing, to avoid feeling like a nuisance… how men seeking access to equipment approached them prior to asking men in the same space, which resulted in some women feeling pressured to finish quickly. Or the men flat out refused or were reluctant to share equipment or space, which led women to abandon an activity."

And well they should stay the **HECK** out of the way when, like Hua, they're so obviously unobservant and outright oblivious to any sense or semblance of universally customary **GYM ETIQUETTE**, aka **GOOD MANNERS, COMMON COURTESY, AND CONSIDERATION!**

So get a **CLUE**, Hua:

Expert exercisers have specific and **TIME**–constrained purposes for going to the gym far beyond, say, intensifying weight–lifting by increasing pound-ages. Maintaining the "muscle pump" by resting just a minute or less between sets is another way of inten-sifying the workout, as is deeply concentrating on all movements performed with intense focus. These are the most basic of training concepts which the inexpe-rienced and workout–*INCOMPETENT* can and nev-er would understand or comprehend. These are well–founded reasons why inept and runty little girls like Hua *DO* pose a decidedly detrimental *NUISANCE* while they're standing on top of the weight rack to watch themselves in the mirror perform their slug-gish little sets of low–impact, low–resistance exercise "lifting" their three–to–five–pound dumbbells for a lengthy 12–15 repetitions!

Expert exercisers on strict workout *SCHED-ULES*, you see, aspire to excel and attain superior levels of development and improvement—being nei-ther complacent about mal–practicing the self–delud-ing *ILLUSION* of working out nor content with me-diocre or inferior accomplishment!

"Hence the crowds of mostly women in cardio classes and mostly men in the weight room," Hua wit-lessly concludes. *"Sounds we could all benefit from crossing over, to put ourselves in someone else's shoes, to treat others as we want to be treated, one workout at a time."*

Quite the contrary, Hua: don't presume, so prema-turely, that your ill–qualified little self is so *SELF*–entitled that "crossing over" will *EVER* "benefit" anybody until you *FIRST* learn how to train *COR-RECTLY* and know what the *HECK* you're doing be-fore so *OBNOXIOUSLY* invading and disrupting the workout space of those accomplished and competent experts who already do!

STAY FIT(AND HOT)FOR LIFE

www.ingramcontent.com/pod-product-compliance
Lightning Source LLC
Chambersburg PA
CBHW031507270326
41930CB00006B/285